Stop Counting Calories & Start Losing Weight

The Harcombe Diet

First published in the US by Create Space 2010

ISBN 1449925723

Copyright © Zoë Harcombe 2008

Zoë Harcombe has asserted her right to be identified as
the author of this work in accordance with the
Copyright, Designs and Patents Act 1988.

Cover design by Lewis Kokoc

The advice offered in this book, although based on the
author's experience and over twenty years of research, is not
intended to be a substitute for the advice of your personal
physician. Always consult a medical practitioner before
embarking on any diet. Neither the author nor the publisher
can be held responsible for any loss or claim arising from the
use or misuse of this book.

Thank You...

Thank you readers of *Why do you overeat? When all you want is to be slim* and the first edition of *Stop Counting Calories & Start Losing Weight*, for your emails, letters, testimonials and questions. You've provided many of the Questions & Answers in Part 6 and your weight loss and better health stories have made it all worth-while.

Thank you Larry, Simone and Brianna for making me feel that a little help can make a big difference.

Thank you Andy for all that you are and for all that you help me to be.

Stop Counting Calories & Start Losing Weight

The Harcombe Diet

This is some of the feedback from people who have tried, and loved, The Harcombe Diet:

"I was so excited just reading the back cover – this was me! I lost 7lb in the first 10 days without feeling hungry at all."

"For the first time in my life I know I will be slim. I have started the programme, I'm not hungry, the cravings have gone and I know how to stop them coming back. The feeling of liberation is indescribable."

"I lost 70lb on this programme. It was easy to follow. I never felt hungry. I could eat out, take lunches to work, go on holiday and carry on with my normal life whilst still losing weight. It is so practical and effective. All my colleagues were asking me how I had lost so much weight and I actually didn't want to tell them. I wanted to keep the secret to myself!"

"I've changed my weighing day to Wednesday and last night I had lost 14.5lb – my first stone!!! This weight loss has been ENTIRELY due to you and your wonderful book. It gave me an understanding and has made this weight loss extremely easy ... it is an awesome thought to know that I shall continue to lose weight thanks to minor changes in my diet. So my sincere thanks, it is doing wonders for my self esteem and life has never been so exciting and challenging."

"I have been following your diet for the last 4 days and have lost 5lb! It was a real struggle not to eat sweet things but my willpower held out. Am looking forward to starting Phase 2 to see what happens."

"I've lost 8lb in 4 days! I can't believe it. I didn't even feel ill like the book said I might. I feel great. I did have huge cravings for sugar for the first couple of days but I didn't give in and I'm really glad I didn't."

"I started Phase 1 and after 2 days I had lost 5lb. I actually thought the scales were wrong but I got on the next day and I had definitely lost 5lb. I had just finished an 8 week programme with a personal trainer and I didn't lose a single pound and I was so demotivated. Then I tried this for 2 days and lost 5lb. It was incredible!"

"I'm on day 3 of Phase 1 and it's going really well. I don't feel as ill as I thought I would, I have been going to bed early to make the evening temptation time shorter but it's worth it 'cos I've lost half a stone already."

"Thank you for writing such a wonderful book. You explain it so well!!!"

"I have been doing your diet for the last three weeks and it's brilliant! I have lost lots of weight and feel in control of my eating with no cravings at all. In fact, I feel like a different person. I have lots more energy and feel much happier in myself because of all the benefits."

"I started your book last night – and finished it a few hours later! You didn't tell me it would be compulsive! I kept reading about all these things that I knew something about and you pieced them altogether. It made so much sense! I don't need to lose more than a couple of pounds but I do need more energy and I'm sure this Candida thing is a big problem for me. Phase 1 here I come!"

"I just wanted to say how pleased I am already. I have read the whole book, done the 5-day kick start programme and have lost 5lb. I can't believe it!"

"I bought your book just over a fortnight ago and I'm impressed!! I followed Phase 1 for the 5 days and lost 8lbs and have now moved onto Phase 2..."

"I just couldn't wait to call everyone this morning. I was at mum's last night and weighed myself as we don't have scales at home. I knew I'd lost a lot of weight but I found out I've lost 24lb – nearly 2st! In under a month. I just can't believe it. I've been telling everyone (not that I need to because they can see for themselves!) I feel great too – I can't remember feeling better to be honest. Thank you so much for the diet!"

"I lost 5lb in Phase 1 and I've lost 10lb altogether in the first 2 weeks. Everyone at work wants a copy of your book because they hadn't seen me for a week and didn't recognise me when I got back! I feel fantastic too – more energy than ever. My skin is so clear – I just look so well – not just slimmer. Thank you so much."

"I feel like I've got a secret that no one else knows – the secret of how to lose weight! I lost 7lb in Phase 1 and a stone in the first 2 weeks. I socialise a lot so I need to 'cheat' when I'm out and this diet actually tells me how to do that. I have my beer and dinner out but I don't go mad. This is just fantastic!"

"I have every one of the conditions in the book and then some. I have been bed ridden for several days in the past few months. Phase 1 nearly finished me off but I knew why I felt so bad. I just kept thinking of the word 'parasite' and it kept me going. I was so determined I didn't know what had come over me. At the end of Phase 1, I felt incredible. I've been waking at 5.30am with an energy I have never known. I feel clear headed. Until I started this plan I could not remember a day when I had not had chocolate and now I haven't had it for weeks. I just don't crave food any more. I'm loving doing things around the house and the garden with all this energy I now have. I can't thank you enough."

"I have been meaning to update you on my progress since reading your book. By the way I enjoyed the book so much I read it twice!!!! First book I have read in years. I have lost 10 pounds in 3 weeks so I am over the moon! I am going for 2 stone total loss to get to my ideal weight. Thanks for writing the book I have recommended it to lots of family and friends."

"I feel that this is the best healthy eating plan I've tried and I never feel hungry."

"I'm so tired today from having stayed up to read your book last night. I couldn't put it down! It makes so much sense and I feel like you're standing here reading it to me when I'm going through it. It's like having a personal coach!"

"I just love your book. I'm training for a marathon and have always struggled with sugar highs and lows. I'm following the Phase 2 advice and eating the most enormous quantities you can imagine and I am staying at the right weight and finding the training is going so well. The advice just makes so much sense. My health is so important to me so I really like the idea of nourishing my body with only good foods."

"Zoë, I am going to get there, thanks to you. I couldn't believe my eyes when I weighed this morning – I've lost a phenomenal 10lb already and this is only the beginning of Day 4! What's more, no hunger cravings whatsoever. What joy to find a route back to a normal size – thanks once again for being caring and generous to share your findings and research."

"What an Easter present – both my partner and I have lost 10lb in 9 days – this is the fastest weight loss we have ever experienced – even more than on Atkins. What's more we feel great! We're sleeping well, the cravings have gone, we feel clear headed and just alive really. Thank you so much."

"Just thought I'd drop you a line to say that I am extremely impressed; I've lost half a stone since Friday and my trousers are falling down (could be a bit embarrassing really)! Here's to the next 6.5st! Thank you ever so much – the book is such an inspiration – my mum is going on it too."

"I'm doing brilliantly – 10lb in 2 weeks and 1 week of that was on holiday. I found it surprisingly easy to stick to on holiday – tropical fruits for breakfast one day and meat, cheese and omelette the next. The fat meals were dead easy for main meals and I just wasn't hungry. I even cheated with quite a lot of alcohol and I still lost weight."

"I am just emailing to thank you for your book! A month or so ago, I did the 5-day plan and lost 7 pounds! Admittedly, I felt awful for the majority of those 5 days, I was v pleased with the results. I've previously tried both Weight Watchers and Slimming World diets and food plans, but couldn't handle being able to eat 'whatever I liked, but in moderation': I can never stand to leave things half-eaten or just take tiny portions of food I love!"

"At last I have found an eating plan that really works for me. I have struggled for the last 8 years trying to diet without much success, in that I lose the weight but always put on more than I lost. I only hope that Phase 2 will get me back down to my natural weight, closer to what I was like 7 years ago when I met my husband."

"I don't know if you remember me or not but I just wanted to say "thank you for changing my life". Since I last sent you an email I have gone down two dress sizes and my cravings have completely gone... Anyway, once again, thanks so much for writing that book and getting me out of my rollercoaster!"

"I have just finished my Phase I of your diet and have lost 6 pounds. I feel absolutely wonderful and have loads of energy. On to Phase 2 now!! Thank you so much."

"Thank goodness someone put all the diet books, eating plans and explanations as to why the other diets don't work into one book and in plain English. Thanks."

"This seems so unfair! I am now at my ideal weight and I love fitting into all my clothes and yet I can eat chocolate, ice cream, just about anything I want and maintain this weight. I've become a complete cheating connoisseur (as this book explains) and I get away with whatever I can."

"Hubby has lost 9lb now in 2 weeks – he hasn't even really been trying! And he hasn't even read the book – he just phones me up and says 'can I have this?' and I say 'yes' or 'no'. Men!"

"I started Phase one on Monday it is only Friday tea-time and I have lost 8lbs - I am absolutely delighted! I am looking forward to losing a few more pounds to see the real benefit in my clothes. I have tried various diets but to be honest this is the one which I have managed to stick to without cheating at all - so that in itself is an achievement for me. Thanks for writing this book – it is fab."

"I need this book! The person who recommended it is literally fading away in front of my eyes but he's bouncing around with energy like Tigger – what has happened to him?!"

"Thank you for such an excellent book! I do believe it is life changing! I'm in Australia and have been battling with Candida for the last few months. I've altered my diet after reading your book... Again many, many thanks for showing me the road to recovery."

"I have been following your plan for 3 weeks now, and I am on Phase 2. No cravings, my wheat intolerance is under control, and my blood sugar cravings have stopped! I have just ordered my 3rd book – the second was for a close friend, and I have just ordered 1 for a friend in France. I think your book is the best thing to happen to me for the last 26years. I have been counting calories and eating low fat thinking I was doing right, and losing and putting on weight all these years! Lost 47lbs with weight watchers, and put 20lbs back on, have thrown all their products away!"

"Brilliant book! My husband and I have been dieting following your instructions in the book and we are really doing well."

"Praise be for you and your book!!! I have just read it from cover to cover and identified so strongly with it that, at times I was moved to tears...in a very positive way of course! Never has text jumped up from the page and screamed, 'this is you.....you don't have to go on like this!' I can now see that I have been equipped with the knowledge to work towards that very slim and shiny Holy Grail! For many years I have struggled with my weight...moving in ever decreasing circles on each new calorie counting expedition. I sought help for my low self esteem, addressed the issues of comfort eating, to little or no avail and you know how destructive this is. Now the 'light' has gone on in my head and for the first time in my adult life I can actually see a way out. Thanks for that!"

"Just a big THANK YOU for writing your book, and therefore helping me! I have struggled since 14 (now 38) with anorexia, bulimia and then just straight forward overeating/compulsive eating and thought all this time it was just my lack of willpower."

"Your book is amazing!"

"I just wanted to say a big thank you for your brilliant book, it really made sense to me. Just finished Phase 1 and I feel great! No cravings at all even when my husband eats chocolate in front of me…! I was really scared to weigh myself this morning just in case I hadn't lost weight as I didn't want to be demoralised if the scales didn't reflect how I was feeling, but guess what?...I lost 7 pounds in 5 days and I feel fantastic and motivated to carry on. Many many thanks, Phase 2 here I come!"

"I have read your super book and followed your eating plan and was amazed at the speed of the weight loss. I lost 9lbs. in the 5 days. I felt much brighter and strangely I felt my eye sight was better and sharper and food actually tasted better after the 5 days. I have never believed in diets and never had a problem with my weight and I wasn't overweight but I was addicted to sugar. When I read your book, it appealed to me, the fact that you could eat well and still lose weight and rid myself of the craving for sugar. Many thanks for writing such a sensible book."

"I am on day 5 of the induction week. Going well, I have lost 9lbs! Where were you when I was 17 and podgy! Thank goodness you're here to see me at 34 and hopefully slim! I believe I am going to do it this time. The book is fab and actually makes a lot of sense."

"I read 4 pages and lost two and a half stone – I figured I'd better not read much more!"

"This is the book I should have written!" (Quote from a Nutritionist, Counsellor, Hypnotherapist & Homeopath).

Contents

Testimonials

Part 1 – Headlines (p1)

1   - How did The Harcombe Diet come about?

     - What is The Harcombe Diet?

     - How is this different to other diets?

     - What can I eat on The Harcombe Diet?

     - How much will I lose?

     - Will I have to exercise?

     - Can I follow this diet as a Vegetarian?

     - Can I follow this diet and still drink alcohol?

     - Who is this book for?

     - How can this book help?

     - Why have I failed so many times before?

     - Why will I succeed this time?

Part 2 – Stop Counting Calories & Start Losing Weight (p27)

2   - What is overweight? Am I overweight?

     - What is "The Obesity Epidemic?"

     - What is the current advice to fix this?

     - Where does calorie counting come from?

     - Does this calorie counting theory work?

     - What happens when we count calories?

     - Stop counting calories & start losing weight

Part 3 – The 3 Medical Conditions, which make you overeat (p49)

3 Candida

4 Food Intolerance

5 Hypoglycaemia

- What is each condition?

- What causes it?

- How do I know if I've got it?

- How does it cause food cravings?

- How can I treat it?

Part 4 – The Harcombe Diet (p97)

6 Phase 1 & Menu plans

7 Phase 2 & Menu plans

8 Phase 3 & Menu plans

- What can I eat?

- How long is each phase?

- When do I eat?

- How much do I eat?

- Why does it work?

- How will I feel?

Part 5 – Psychological Factors (p169)

9   Eating disorders – my personal story

10 Eating disorders generally

11 Why do we overeat?

12 How to overcome the diet destroying voices in your head

Part 6 – Questions & Answers (p205)

- The Top 10 Frequently Asked Questions
- The Harcombe Diet vs. traditional diet advice
- Candida, Food Intolerance & Hypoglycaemia
- Cravings
- Specific foods
- Carbs, fats, protein and mixing
- Shopping
- Drinks
- Medical considerations
- Personal Questions

Part 7 – Recipes (p293)

Part 8 – Appendices (p329)

1 – Glossary of Terms
2 – Recommended Reading
3 – Vitamins & Minerals Tables

About the Author

Index

Part 1

Headlines

1

Headlines

How did The Harcombe Diet come about?

The Harcombe Diet came about as the result of:

1) Twenty years' worth of research into diets, diet advice, the characteristics of a 'workable' diet, obesity, eating disorders, food cravings and what causes them;

2) The author's own experience of dieting, eating disorders, unworkable diets, food cravings and what causes them; and

3) The author's determination to answer the question *"Why do people overeat, when they want so badly to be slim"?*

I have huge faith in people and our ability to achieve what we want to. I don't think we are (generally) greedy, weak-willed, lazy, or all the other horrible labels that are given to overweight people. I believe that, if someone wants to be slim, more than they want anything else, nothing would logically stand in the way of that goal.

This was my own experience, as I sat in my college room at Cambridge University, stuffing my face with food. I'm a bright girl, I thought. I am not enjoying this binge. I hate the fact that it is ruining my diet and it is going to make me fat. Why, on earth, am I doing this? Also – how come I never binge on brown rice and stir-fry vegetables? What is the unique attraction of confectionery, biscuits, cakes, bread and crisps?!

I came to the conclusion that, for someone to **not** be able to stick to a diet, when they want so much to be able to stick to it, there must be something else going on. There must be something wrecking our willpower, causing these addict-like cravings, otherwise we would stick to the diet and achieve our dreams. What on earth could it be?

That question, and the research that followed, led to three conclusions:

1) First of all, the diet advice we have been given is fundamentally wrong. I am absolutely convinced that telling people to "*eat less, do more*" is the **cause** of the obesity problem, not the cure. This book will explain exactly what happens, directly and indirectly, when we try to eat less and how our bodies will work against us to keep us alive and sabotage any attempts to lose weight.

2) The second huge discovery was that there are three medical conditions, which cause insatiable food cravings. These three conditions are extremely common – you probably suffer from at least one of them, if not all three. If you do suffer from any of them, they each cause food cravings in their own destructive way and you will have no chance of sticking to a diet until you overcome them.

3) The final shock discovery was that, if you have ever counted calories, or tried to eat less, you have substantially increased your chance of having one, or more of these conditions. That means – your previous attempts to diet have almost certainly given you the three medical conditions that will turn you into a food addict!

So – go on a low calorie/low fat/eat less kind of diet and your body will do everything it can to wreck your diet and you will be highly likely to develop three medical conditions that will give you addict-like cravings to further wreck your diet. No wonder the more I tried to starve the more I ended up bingeing!

Just quickly, we'll do fact boxes on each of these three conditions – because they will be referred to throughout the book from now on.

We use fact boxes occasionally in the book, just to explain a key 'fact' that is helpful to know. There is also a Glossary of Terms, at the back of the book, so that you can check any definition any time you come across it in the book. The Glossary has the following definitions for Candida, Food Intolerance and Hypoglycaemia, as well as definitions for Insulin, Blood Glucose Level and other useful terms.

In Part 3 of the book, these three conditions will be fully explained – what are they? What causes them? How do you know if you've got them? How do you get rid of them?

Here are the headlines for now:

Fact Box: Candida is a yeast, which lives in all of us, and is normally kept under control by our immune system and other bacteria in our body. It usually lives in the digestive system. Candida has no useful purpose. If it stays quiet and in balance, it causes no harm. The problem starts if Candida multiplies out of control and then it can create havoc with our health and wellbeing. Candida has been shown to cause insatiable food cravings – particularly for all sugary foods, bread, cakes, biscuits, fruit/fruit juices and vinegary/pickled foods.

Fact Box: Food Intolerance means, quite simply, not being able to tolerate a particular food. This is different to Food Allergy – Food Allergy is the really serious, life threatening, condition where people have nut, or strawberry allergies, for example. Food Intolerance develops when you have too much of a food and too often and your body just gets to the point where it can't cope with that food any longer. Food Intolerance can also make a person feel horribly unwell. The real irony is that Food Intolerance causes people to crave the foods to which they are intolerant. You are most likely to be intolerant to anything you have daily and feel you couldn't live without.

Fact Box: Hypoglycaemia is literally a Greek translation from "*hypo*" meaning 'under', "*glykis*" meaning 'sweet' and "*emia*" meaning 'in the blood together'. The three bits all put together mean low blood sugar. Hypoglycaemia describes the state your body is in if your blood sugar levels are too low. When your blood sugar levels are too low, this is potentially life threatening and your body will try to get you to eat. Hypoglycaemia can cause cravings for any carbohydrate – even fruit.

What is The Harcombe Diet?

The Harcombe Diet has used all this research to come up with a diet that overcomes these problems. It is designed to **not** make you hungry and to **not** have you craving food. This means that you can stick to it and start losing weight.

The Harcombe Diet has three Phases:

Phase 1 (just five days long) is designed to do the following:

- To 'kick-start' your new way of eating with a programme that is short enough to stick to, but long enough to have a significant impact on Candida, Food Intolerance and Hypoglycaemia;

- To attack food cravings head on (by attacking Candida, Food Intolerance and Hypoglycaemia head on) when motivation and willpower are highest, at the start of a new diet;

- To achieve significant weight loss.

Phase 2 (for as long as you want to lose weight) is designed to do the following:

- To continue to win the war against Candida, Food Intolerance and Hypoglycaemia (and so to have continued impact on food cravings);

- To continue the great start made in Phase 1, but with a more varied diet, which is more enjoyable;

- To change your eating habits forever. To get you eating real food and nourishing your body and to put you off processed foods and 'junk' as much as possible.

Phase 3 (for as long as you want to maintain your weight) is designed to do the following:

- To put you back in control of your eating by giving you long-term control over food cravings;

- To enable you to eat, without cravings, for life;
- To enable you to eat whatever you want, **almost** whenever you want, but with you managing the outcome.

The Harcombe Diet – what it **doesn't** do:

- It does not count calories, or carbohydrates, or fat units, or points – it does not count anything;
- It does not limit quantities of food;
- It does not put your life on hold while you lose weight;
- It does not come with, nor need, an exercise plan;
- It does not try to get you to eat less and do more.

The Harcombe Diet – what it **does** do:

- It defines and meets all the characteristics of a successful diet;
- It lets you eat real food in unlimited quantities;
- It gives you three simple rules, to lose weight and stay slim for life;
- It encourages you to work with your body, not against it;
- It lets you get on with your life and eat to live, not live to eat.

I've been asked by journalists – if you don't agree with the "*Eat less, do more*" advice – what do you agree with? My answer is "*Eat better and do whatever you like*".

I've also been asked – is the diet low carb or low fat and the answer is neither. It is good carbs and good fats – in whatever quantities you want – just not at the same meal.

How is this different to other diets?

Almost every other diet is trying to get you to eat less. Some also have an exercise plan, to get you to do more. Any calorie-counted diet; any low fat diet; any points diet (Weight Watchers ®); any fad diet – all of these are trying to get you to eat less. You are going to see in Part 2 that trying to eat less is disastrous for your body and your weight loss attempts.

Atkins, and other very low carbohydrate diets, are in a different category – they try to get you to avoid carbohydrates, but they don't restrict your calories. You will see that I am a bigger fan of low carbohydrate diets, than I am of low calorie diets, but you don't have to do either to lose weight...

The five characteristics of a successful diet are:

1) It must work – and not just in the short term. It must help you reach your natural weight and stay there.

2) It must be practical – a real diet for the real world. No working out grams of protein or counting calories or carbohydrates – some simple rules that you can follow at home, at work or eating out, as part of your busy lifestyle.

3) It must be something you can follow for life – a real lifestyle change – something you can stick to easily and not something you go on and then go off leading to life-long weight fluctuations.

4) It must be healthy – and deliver the nutrients you need for healthy living.

5) It must be enjoyable – and not take away eating as a pleasure in life.

The Harcombe Diet meets all of the above criteria and I am not aware of another diet that does.

If we look at diets, which you may have tried so far, they all fall down in one or more areas. There is a summary below. (Please note this is my own interpretation from experience and research – you may have found *The Cabbage Soup Diet* most enjoyable, for example, so you can add your own ticks and crosses). The chances are, if you have found one of these to work for you in the long term, you won't be reading this book anyway.

	Fad diet	Low Carb diet	Low calorie diet	The Harcombe Diet
It works long term	✗	✓ (1)	✗	✓
It's practical	✗	✗	✓	✓
It's a lifestyle change	✗	✓ (1)	✗/✓	✓
It's healthy	✗	✗/✓	✗	✓
It's enjoyable	✗	✗/✓	✗/✓	✓

Note (1) – if you can stick to it.

Fad Diets

As you can see with fad diets, they have nothing to recommend them – they work in the short term but may well contribute to weight gain in the long term as you slow down your metabolism, lose lean muscle and do other long term damage. They are rarely practical and require you to eat alone, avoid all social events and put your life on hold while you are on the diet. They cannot be followed in the long term. They are not healthy, as they usually tell you to eat one food, or very few foods, to the exclusion of all others, and they are rarely enjoyable.

Low Carbohydrate Diets

Low carbohydrate diets, like the Atkins Diet, can work, and they can work in the long term, if you can stick to them. The key is if you can stick to them, of course. They also work quite well with cravings, as they tend to cut out foods that cause Candida, Food Intolerance and Hypoglycaemia. However, they miss out on the practical side of things, as it just isn't possible to have shrimps in butter, or steak, at your office desk.

In terms of whether or not they are enjoyable I think this varies by person. For a carnivore, that loves the idea of animals at each meal, they may be enjoyable but they are virtually impossible for Vegetarians and they don't allow enough variety and flexibility for many to enjoy this diet.

I actually think that they are far healthier than many reports suggest. Very low carbohydrate diets have been linked to heart disease, kidney damage, osteoporosis, halitosis (bad breath), cataracts, muscle weakness, asthma and constipation. However, for an estimated 3.5 million years, the major part of the human diet (and that of our ancestors) has been animals and their by products, so I struggle to believe the health scares linked to low carb diets. Bad breath, maybe, but heart disease – I really don't think so.

The bottom line is that you don't need to go this far to lose weight and stay slim forever. You can eat steak and salad, as these diets encourage, but you can also eat brown pasta and stir-fry, fruit and a much wider variety of food and still lose weight.

Low Calorie Diets

Low calorie diets ironically score quite well against most criteria, except that they don't work in the long run. They are practical – mostly people eat 'normal' foods, but just less of them. People can eat cereal for breakfast, fruit for snacks, calorie counted sandwiches for lunch, calorie counted ready cooked meals for dinner and perhaps a calorie counted 'treat' somewhere during the day. The big problem is that people can't stick to them, because they get so hungry and because these diets lead to conditions that cause food cravings (we will see exactly how).

Calorie controlled diets can be moderately healthy, depending on the foods chosen, but they fall down on being healthy overall as, by definition, you are eating less food than you actually need. They also score a mixed rating for how enjoyable they are, as they do allow you to eat what you want, which is a plus, but they restrict quantities so much that this can't be enjoyable overall.

The main problem is that low calorie diets don't work in the long term. They may work in the short term, and then only if you can stick to them. The problem is that, in the long term, our bodies adjust to the continued starvation and the weight loss slows or even stops altogether. Then, our bodies need less food to survive on a daily basis, so, if we go back to eating the same food we ate before the low calorie diet we will actually put on weight. When we say calorie counting doesn't work, therefore, we are saying that it doesn't work *in the long term*. Calorie counting sends you into a vicious circle of eating less and less just to stay at the same weight.

Let's finish this section looking at some other well-known diets, not in the tick and cross table above...

Low Carbohydrate AND Low Calorie

Some diets are low in carbs and calories. I think *"The Zone"* and the *"South Beach Diet"* fall into this category.

"A Week in the Zone" does say that the total calorie content for a day in the Zone is about 1200 calories. The diet also gets you to count protein blocks and

carbohydrate blocks and limits how many you can have. On The Zone diet I would be 'allowed' 10 carbohydrate blocks, which would be used up with "*one 4oz bowl of porridge oats made with 2 cups of milk.*" I then wouldn't be able to have any more carbs for the rest of the day.

The South Beach diet adds up to approximately 1200-1500 calories per day. The first fourteen days are extremely low carb – no carrots, let alone the rice we can have in our Phase 1. After this fortnight, more carbs are allowed, but The South Beach Diet is still described as 'a low carb diet' when people write about it. I analysed the carbs in the menu plans for 'Phase 2' and they seemed to add up to barely 50g of carbohydrate on some days (e.g. Day 5) and as many as 200g on other days (e.g. Day 6).

If we look at diets that are low carbohydrate and low calorie, against the five characteristics of a successful diet, in some ways they mix the worst of both diets. They don't let you have unlimited amounts of meat, fish eggs and cheese, as low carb diets do. (Having fruit and other carbs may well compensate for this). However, given that low carb and low calorie diets restrict calories, they still get you to eat less than you need. This means that you will still experience all the problems associated with this, which we describe in Part 2. The South Beach looks more practical than The Zone, but there are still up to 7 recipes a day to follow, even in the most 'back to basics' part of the diet.

Low Glycaemic Index (GI) diets

This is the final category of diets worth commenting upon. A low GI diet is one that limits foods with a high Glycaemic Index. The Glycaemic Index is the measure of the effect of any food on blood glucose levels over a period of time. Glucose is the purest substance from which the body can get energy. The index uses the impact of pure glucose being consumed as '100' and then measures all other foods against this. Popcorn has a high Glycaemic Index, approximately 85. Meat has a GI score of 0 – because it has no impact on blood glucose at all.

The GI diet is based on a great fact – and one that this book whole-heartedly endorses – that insulin is what makes you fat and not calories. When you eat any carbohydrate your body produces a hormone, called insulin, to return your blood glucose level back into the safe range. The Glycaemic Index, simply measures how much your blood glucose level is going to rise with each particular food and therefore how much insulin needs to be produced to return your blood glucose level to normal.

> Fact Box: As your blood glucose level rises, insulin is released from the pancreas and this insulin converts some of the glucose to glycogen. (Glycogen is our energy store room). If all the glycogen storage areas are full, insulin will convert the excess to fatty tissue. This is why insulin has been called the fattening hormone.

So, the diet advises, eat foods low on the GI index (generally with a GI of less than 50) and you will naturally manage this blood glucose level mechanism and avoid too much insulin, the fattening hormone, sloshing around your body. This is sound advice and I am quite a fan of GI diets. The big problem with GI diets is that they still let you eat the foods that feed the three medical conditions in this book. You won't get rid of food cravings, and be able to stick to any diet, if you don't get rid of these three conditions.

Specifically with Food Intolerance, the GI diet doesn't lead you to avoid foods to which you could be intolerant. You can still have wheat, for example, and dairy products are actively encouraged. As a particular example, rice has a higher GI than pasta, so people on a low GI diet will be encouraged to eat pasta, rather than rice and rice is far better than pasta for Food Intolerance.

In terms of the characteristics of a successful diet, they fall down a bit on the practical criterion. They still require you to count things, or, at least to be aware of the GI for each food. Glycaemic Index tables also vary quite widely in their scores. I've also seen GI scores for dried fruit, as an example, range from 35 to 60, which is too wide for comfort. If I were going to count anything to try to lose weight, I would want to at least know that it was accurate.

It is helpful, for people doing The Harcombe Diet, to be aware of 'real foods', with a high Glycaemic Index, as these are the ones that you should take care with, if you have Hypoglycaemia. Things like baked potatoes, bananas and even (cooked) carrots, have a high GI score and can therefore be a problem for someone very sensitive to carbohydrates.

OK, so that's a quick run through of all the categories of diets you could have tried to date. Now let's turn to the one that meets all the characteristics of a successful diet...

The Harcombe Diet

The Harcombe Diet meets all the characteristics of a successful diet:

1) Number one, it works and it works long term. Because the diet works with your body, not against it, your body doesn't start trying to fight you and make you eat/crave food.

2) It is practical – no _ grapefruits, no rigid meal times, no complex recipes, no prescribed meals to eat and nothing to count. It just has simple 'dos and don'ts', by which you can manage your own eating, to fit in with your own lifestyle.

3) It is a diet that you can follow for life to help you reach and stay at your natural weight.

4) It is healthy and nutritious – it gives you the vitamins and minerals you need for optimal health. It also advises that you avoid processed foods, which do little, if anything, for your health and nutrition.

5) It is enjoyable. It frees you from cravings and lets you eat when you are hungry and when your body needs food. It allows as wide a variety of food as possible and allows 'treats' as often as your body can cope with them, once you have reached your natural weight.

The Harcombe Diet is the first diet to directly and indirectly explain cravings – why you get them, what causes them, what impact calorie controlled diets have on them and how to get rid of them. It is also the first book to directly link Candida, Food Intolerance and Hypoglycaemia with food cravings (all of these will be explained in Part 3).

What can I eat on The Harcombe Diet?

Phase 1 lasts for just five days and you can eat meat, fish, eggs, vegetables and salads (except potatoes and mushrooms), brown rice (in moderation) and Natural Live Yoghurt. Other than the brown rice, quantities are **UN**limited. You can go back to Phase 1 at any time and you will have a five-day plan with you, for life, which can lose you up to 14 pounds in less than a week.

Example meals would be bacon and eggs for breakfast; Salade Niçoise for lunch and butternut squash curry and brown rice for dinner.

Phase 2 should be followed for as long as you need to lose weight. It can be followed for life, as it is healthy, enjoyable and easy to follow. You will be able to eat any real food – steak, seafood, fruit, baked potatoes, (wholemeal) pasta, (wholemeal) bread, and cheese. You will even be able to enjoy (red) wine and dark chocolate on occasions.

There are just 3 rules:

1) Don't eat processed foods;

2) Don't eat fats and carbohydrates at the same meal;

3) Don't eat foods that cause **your** cravings.

All of the rules will be explained simply and clearly so you will know exactly what is a fat meal and a carbohydrate meal and which food(s) you particularly need to avoid. The simplicity and power of the above rules may fascinate you. You will learn why avoiding processed foods alone will transform your weight loss attempts. You will soon learn how the body uses food and how it can only store fat if you eat carbohydrate at the same time and therefore why you should never want to eat carbs and fats together again.

Example meals on The Harcombe Diet would be porridge with skimmed milk for breakfast; wholemeal pita breads with hummus and salad for lunch and smoked salmon starter, steak and vegetables main course and cheese platter for dessert.

Phase 1 and Phase 2 are set out for what I have called "*Flexis*" and "*Planners*". Flexis don't want a prescriptive diet – they want a list of 'do's' and 'don'ts' and a list of suggested meals and they then get on and do their flexi plan. Planners want to know what to have on Monday for breakfast and Tuesday for lunch and they are quite happy for someone to have planned this all out for them. This book caters for both Flexis and Planners, so it can meet the needs of all types of people. Phase 1 and Phase 2 also have Flexi and Planner menu options for Vegetarians.

Phase 3 is about how to have your cake and eat it. Phase 3 takes the principles of Phase 2 and shows you how to 'cheat' so that you can enjoy literally any food without putting on weight.

So, Phase 1 is quite a tough start (not as tough as Atkins though). Then, in Phase 2, you can eat everything from steak to pasta and still enjoy fruit, cheese and all real food. Phase 3 should reassure you that there is **no** food that you will have to give up for life. You will be able to eat anything you like and not put on weight, and you will get all the tips for how you can do this.

How much will I lose?

This will be different for every person. Gender plays a part – men tend to lose weight more easily than women. The more you have to lose the more you will lose.

This book will introduce you to three medical conditions that cause insatiable food cravings. If you have been trying to diet/eat less/count calories – anything like this – for even a few months, let alone years, you probably have at least one of these

17

conditions and these are the reasons why you can't lose weight.

The more conditions you have been suffering from, the more weight you will lose on The Harcombe Diet. Two of the three conditions, in particular, are known to play havoc with water retention so, after just five days on Phase 1, you could lose half a stone, or even more.

The key thing is that you will tend towards your natural weight quickly and safely. You will eat healthy, whole foods that nourish you and you will not be hungry. Some of my case studies have had stones to lose and they have lost stones and kept them off. The record weight loss to date has been 17lb on Phase 1. 10-14lb has been achieved on several occasions.

Will I have to exercise?

The debate on exercise is fascinating. Some people say, "...*if only people did more, they would not be overweight...*" The government in the UK seems to think that we shouldn't be too worried about what our children eat – so long as they are doing lots of exercise, and not playing on computer games, all will be fine.

One of the most brilliant TV programmes I ever watched blew this theory sky high. The programme was called "*30 Minutes*" and it was all about childhood obesity. During the programme there was an experiment where the presenter, Nick Cohen, took a boys' football team from London, England, and split them into three groups. One third of the team were given an apple; another third a bag of crisps and the final group a confectionery bar. The teenagers were then asked to run around an athletics track continuously until they had burned off what they had eaten. The apple group needed to run for 13 minutes to burn off the apple. The crisp group needed to run for 42 minutes to burn off the crisps and the confectionery group needed to run for one hour and five minutes to burn off their item. The presenter explained that, if a child ate a bag of crisps, a confectionery bar, a burger and chips and had a fizzy drink, they would need to run for five hours to burn that off!

In short, exercise alone is not going to solve your weight problem. As the "*30 Minutes*" programme showed, the amount of exercise that you need to do to burn off food is astonishing. Furthermore, exercise actually increases your need for energy/fuel. When you exercise, you need more energy (calories), so you need to be careful that you don't finish doing exercise and find yourself so hungry that you want to eat more than you have just used up.

Please don't think that exercise is a bad thing to do. It is in fact a great thing to do, but it won't solve your weight problem. Exercise tones your body and it makes you feel more energetic and healthier. It has been shown to lift mood, reduce stress and make people feel happier and more positive. Exercise can develop the three main aspects of fitness – strength, stamina and suppleness – all great for your health. You can have fun and meet people doing sport, or joining a gym. There are many good reasons to exercise, but trying to rely on exercise to lose weight is not one of them.

The answer to the question above, therefore, is that you do **not** have to exercise for The Harcombe Diet to work. You should, however, exercise for all the other health benefits it offers.

Can I follow this diet as a Vegetarian?

I was a Vegetarian for about fifteen years. In the last couple of years I have started to eat fish again, so I am now a non-meat eater. I was a Vegetarian because I love animals and couldn't bear the thought of eating them, but my most important personal value is health, so I did have a dilemma. Mostly I am enjoying the health benefits of eating fish. Every now and again I think of the fish swimming around in the sea and I struggle. So, I can understand that eating animals is a very emotive and personal subject and it has to be your choice. I really can understand if you can't face eating meat or fish.

If you are suffering from Candida, it will be very difficult for you to overcome this condition whilst being a Vegetarian. It will be close to impossible as a Vegan. As the most basic anti-Candida diet is meat, fish, eggs, salad, vegetables and Natural Live Yoghurt, if you do not eat any animal foods you will not be able to control Candida easily through diet. Vegans would have to live on vegetables to follow the strict anti-Candida diet and this would not be healthy, or give them anywhere near enough energy.

The other problem for Vegetarians is that there are only two zero carb food groups – meat and fish – and Vegetarians don't eat these. Hence everything that Vegetarians eat has some carbohydrate. The amount in eggs is negligible, the amount in dairy products is very small (less than 5%), but the amount in fruit and whole grains can be considerable. As carbs cause insulin to be released and insulin is the fattening hormone, Vegetarians will be unlikely to lose weight as quickly and easily as carnivores.

In terms of food options, Vegetarians will find Phase 1 more difficult than meat and fish eaters will, but Phase 1 is only five days long, so it is really not that big a problem. Phase 2 is great for Vegetarians, because, as you will see, all carbohydrate meals are naturally vegetarian.

The bottom line, therefore, is that you can follow this diet and be a Vegetarian. However, if you have a significant problem with Candida you should seriously consider eating fish and/or meat for a period of time, just to get your Candida back under control.

Can I follow this diet and still drink alcohol?

You can't drink alcohol for the first five days – Phase 1. In Phase 2 you can drink occasionally, in moderation, ideally red wine. In Phase 3, you can use your entire 'cheating' on alcohol, if you wish.

If you are concerned that you may be an alcoholic as well as a food addict, this book could change your life. The principles in this book have huge relevance for people suffering from alcoholism. Alcoholics are not greedy or weak-willed. They are suffering an addiction, just like smokers, drug addicts and food addicts.

A critical thing to note about alcoholism is that an alcoholic may feel addicted to *drinking* alcohol, as a habit, but physically they are almost certainly addicted to the ingredients in alcohol rather than alcohol as a pure substance (ethanol) or as a category of drinks. A food addict, with an addiction to wheat, craves biscuits, cakes, pasta, bread and so on. However, they are craving the wheat in biscuits, cakes, pasta and bread and not necessarily the other ingredients. If a wheat addict gives up pasta (which is clearly wheat and not much else), but continues to eat biscuits, they will continue to feed their addiction to wheat and will continue to crave wheat. I suggest that the alcoholic who craves alcohol is actually craving the ingredients in alcohol and not just the general category of alcohol itself. This is hugely significant.

The alcoholic is advised to go 'cold turkey' and to cut out all alcohol, but what if it is the ingredients in alcohol that are being craved? In this situation the alcoholic may stop drinking alcohol, but they may still be consuming the ingredients that they are addicted to on a daily, if not almost hourly, basis. The key ingredients in alcohol are sugar, yeast, grains and concentrated fruit sugar. These are some of the most commonly craved foods and this book will help you understand why.

The other enormous implication of this approach is that alcoholics may not need to give up alcohol forever. If they free themselves of their addiction to the **ingredients** in alcohol, they may be able to drink alcohol again in the future provided that they don't drink too much, or too often. If they return to drinking alcohol in significant quantities every day they will have problems again very quickly. However, if they don't drink too much, or too often, they may be able to return to the social drinking that they were once able to enjoy before the addiction took hold.

So, you won't be able to drink alcohol in Phase 1. The occasional glass of red wine is the best option in Phase 2 and you can do what you want in Phase 3. But, guess what, by Phase 3, having overcome your addiction to things like sugar and wheat, you may well find that your cravings for alcohol have also disappeared.

Who is this book for?

This book is for anyone who wants to lose weight. It is especially for those who want to lose weight so desperately that they can't think what they would like more than this.

It is for anyone who doesn't need to lose weight, but who wants to stop feeling addicted to, and controlled by, food. Perhaps someone who can only maintain his or her current weight by eating small amounts, who wants to be able to eat normally again, without putting on weight.

It is for anyone (often male) who doesn't have 'food problems', but who want to lose weight quickly and easily without making too many sacrifices and whilst being able to get on with their lives at the same time.

It is for anyone who can't stick to a diet – especially for those who can't understand why.

It is for anyone who has ever calorie counted, lost weight, put weight back on and/or put more back on than they first lost.

It is for anyone who found Atkins worked for them, but can't bear the thought of having to avoid fruit, chocolate, bread and the 'good things in life' forever.

It is for anyone who has food cravings, or feels that they are addicted to food in some way. It is especially for people who have particular food cravings – for chocolate, bread, cereal, even salad dressing – all of these will be completely explained.

It is for anyone who experiences unwelcome symptoms after meals – anything from bloating to feeling 'foggy'. It is for anyone whose waistband feels unnaturally uncomfortable after eating.

Whatever type, above, you are, this book is for you. This book can help even the most extreme food addict understand why they crave food and it can help them overcome that addiction. It can help any of you lose weight and it can help you feel so much healthier at the same time. It can help you lose weight and keep it off, with as little deprivation and sacrifice as we can manage.

How can this book help?

By telling you the one thing that you are doing to virtually guarantee you will overeat. That is – counting calories/eating less than you need.

By telling you about three extremely common medical conditions, which are the cause of your overeating. They are Candida, Food Intolerance and Hypoglycaemia.

By helping you identify which of these conditions may be a problem for you and how you overcome them.

By explaining how calorie counting/eating less has got you to where you are today.

By giving you the chance to eat to live rather than living to eat.

By giving you a life-long eating plan which will help you:

- Lose weight and keep the weight off;

- Overcome cravings for good;

- Gain energy and better health;

- Get on with your life, rather than calorie counting all day long.

Why have I failed so many times before?

Because what you have been doing so far has been the **cause** of your weight problem. It will never be the cure. Part 2 will show what happens when you try to eat less/count calories and how you will turn yourself into a food addict – not a successful dieter. Counting calories will lead your body to do the exact opposite of what you want it to, at every stage of the way. This is why you have failed before. It hasn't been your fault at all.

Your body has been working against you, not with you. As soon as you have tried to eat less, your body has tried to get you to eat more. It has made you hungry, it has stored fat and used up your lean muscle and it has reduced your metabolism. All of these things have acted directly against your weight loss efforts.

On top of these direct things that happen, when you try to eat less than you need, indirectly your body has been laid wide open to develop three extremely common medical conditions, which cause insatiable food cravings. These cravings have then made sure that it is near on impossible for you to stick to a diet.

Why will I succeed this time?

Because you will **not** try to eat less, let alone eat less and do more at the same time. By **not** eating less, this alone will make sure that your body works with you and not against you. You are going to experience the immense power of your body working with you, not against you. You are going to nourish and feed yourself with healthy real foods and your body is going to reward you with more energy, better hair and skin and many more benefits.

More importantly, your body will not have to make you hungry, store fat and slow your metabolism down when it sees that it is going to get regular, nutritious meals. It then starts to work with you and it starts to use food/fuel efficiently and you can stick to the healthy diet and finally lose weight.

The final reason why you will succeed this time is because you now have the power of knowledge. You will know why you have failed before – because of the cravings. You will know what you have been craving and why. You will know that the cravings have come from calorie counting, Candida, Food Intolerance and Hypoglycaemia. You will know that you have to eliminate the offending foods from your diet to make the cravings disappear.

Please note...

I use the terms eating less/counting calories interchangeably – because they all amount to the same thing – the *"Eat less, do more"* advice, which doesn't work.

I also use the terms energy/fuel/calories interchangeably – also because they all amount to the same thing. Our bodies need fuel. Another word for fuel is energy and the energy that the body uses is called calories.

When I use the word diet, I don't mean eating less – although this is probably what you have come to think of as a diet. The word diet actually means *"one's habitual food"* – that means – what someone eats on a daily basis. When we talk about the Mediterranean diet, we mean olives, fish, vegetables and so on. The Harcombe Diet describes what you will eat on a daily basis, but it doesn't mean you will eat less.

Part 2

Stop Counting Calories & Start Losing Weight...

2

Stop Counting Calories & Start Losing Weight

What is overweight? Am I overweight?

The general measurement that is now used to define 'overweight' is called the Body Mass Index (BMI). This is a measure of body fat based on height and weight that applies to both men and women. It is calculated by taking a person's weight in kilograms and dividing this by their height in metres squared, e.g. a 70kg person with a height of 1.8m has a Body Mass Index (BMI) of 70/(1.8x1.8) = 21.6. This is in the normal range.

The guidelines are:

- A BMI of less than 18.5 is considered *"Underweight"*;

- A BMI of 18.5 – 24.9 is considered *"Normal"*;

- A BMI of 25 – 29.9 is considered *"Overweight"*;

- A BMI of 30 or more is considered *"Obese"*.

Please note that the Body Mass Index (BMI) calculator is a guide only. It takes no account of muscle vs. fat for example. Using the BMI scale, many athletes, and almost all rugby or American Football players, are classified as overweight. Please use your common sense when applying this calculator – if you are an athlete or an ex-athlete you will know if you are a solid human being, or a flabby one needing some attention.

You can use this BMI calculation to see if you are overweight. Or, you can go on the Internet and enter *"BMI calculator"* and this can do the calculation for you (I have a calculator on my web site: *www.theharcombediet.com*). Or, you can use the Body Mass Index table in this section. This has been converted to inches and pounds, from metres and kilograms, just so that you have both options.

In the table, find your height in inches along the left hand side and then move your finger along that row until you come to your current weight. Look at the number at the top of that column and that will tell you your current BMI. For example, I am 5ft 2in and I weigh 8st (112lb) so I find the row with 62 inches and I am then in the range 109 to 115lb so my BMI is somewhere between 20 and 21. The healthy range is 18.5-24.9 so I am in the middle of the healthy range.

You can then use the chart to see where your weight should be. If you are 5ft 6in (66 inches), your healthy weight will be somewhere in the range 118-148lb. This is a large range, but it allows for both genders and for all different frame sizes.

Please note that I talk about "A natural weight" throughout the book and this is the weight your body will reach at the end of Phase 2 i.e. when you are eating natural, healthy, real foods in the quantities that you need to avoid feeling hungry. It will be the weight that you find you can stay at easily, provided that you don't cheat too much or too often. You will only tend to dip below your natural weight if you are ill and genuinely lose your appetite. You will go above it if you cheat too much, too often.

If you are 5ft, 4in and you want to be 100lb, this is not a healthy goal and this will not be your natural weight. You may, however, find that 115-120lb is a natural weight range for you and you will be a slim, 'small clothes size', person at this weight. Don't be unrealistic with your goal weight, therefore, and don't think too much about your weight as you embark on this programme. The key goal is to stop cravings and doing this will stop the overeating and your weight will then tend towards its natural level quickly and easily.

Body Mass Index Table

BMI	20	21	22	23	24	25	26	27	28	29	30	35	40
Height (in).	Weight (lb).												
58	96	100	105	110	115	119	124	129	134	138	143	167	191
59	99	104	109	114	119	124	128	133	138	143	148	173	198
60	102	107	112	118	123	128	133	138	143	148	153	179	204
61	106	111	116	122	127	132	137	143	148	153	158	185	211
62	109	115	120	126	131	136	142	147	153	158	164	191	218
63	113	118	124	130	135	141	146	152	158	163	169	197	225
64	116	122	128	134	140	145	151	157	163	169	174	204	232
65	120	126	132	138	144	150	156	162	168	174	180	210	240
66	124	130	136	142	148	155	161	167	173	179	186	216	247
67	127	134	140	146	153	159	166	172	178	185	191	223	255
68	131	138	144	151	158	164	171	177	184	190	197	230	262
69	135	142	149	155	162	169	176	182	189	196	203	236	270
70	139	146	153	160	167	174	181	188	195	202	207	243	278
71	143	150	157	165	172	179	186	193	200	208	215	250	286
72	147	154	162	169	177	184	191	199	206	213	221	258	294
73	151	159	166	174	182	189	197	204	212	219	227	265	302
74	155	163	171	179	186	194	202	210	218	225	233	272	311
75	160	168	176	184	192	200	208	216	224	232	240	279	319
76	164	172	180	189	197	205	213	221	230	238	246	287	328

What is "*The obesity Epidemic*"

In 1993, 13% of women and 16% of men in the UK were obese. In 2004, 24% of both women and men, that is one quarter of people in the UK, were obese (i.e. they had a BMI – Body Mass Index – of more than 30). That means obesity almost doubled in just over 10 years in the UK.

In the US, obesity levels increased from 26% to 33% for women and 21% to 28% for men, in a similar time period.

Currently, world-wide, more than one billion adults are overweight – and at least 300 million of them are clinically obese. Current obesity levels range from below 5% in China, Japan and certain African nations, to over 75% in urban Samoa. But even in relatively low obesity countries, like China, rates are almost 20% in some cities.

Childhood obesity is already at epidemic levels in some areas and on the rise in others. 22 million children under five are estimated to be overweight worldwide. According to the US Surgeon General, the number of overweight children in the USA has doubled and the number of overweight adolescents has trebled since 1980.

The above is all about obesity. If we look at overweight people – those with a BMI of more than 25 – at the time of writing this book, approximately two thirds of people in the UK and the USA are overweight. I say "*at the time of writing*" because this number is only going in one direction – up.

The obesity epidemic is, therefore, the term used to describe the number of, and massive increase in the number of, overweight and obese people in so called 'developed' countries.

Along with obesity, comes obesity related illnesses – like Diabetes, heart disease, high blood pressure, some cancers, immobility, depression and so on. Obesity is putting an incredible strain on our health services. Obesity accounts for 2-6% of total health care costs in several developed countries; some estimates put the figure as high as 7%. The true costs are undoubtedly much greater as not all obesity-related conditions are included in the calculations.

Many people are dying way younger than they should and even more are leading sad, miserable lives, hating the body they are in.

What is the current advice to fix this?

The public health advice in the UK and the advice from the US National Institutes of Health is essentially to "*Eat less, do more.*" Quite specifically, the dietary advice from the British Dietetic Association (BDA) is:

"*One pound of fat contains 3500 calories, so to lose 1lb a week you need a deficit of 500 calories a day.*"

The advice from the American Department of Health and Human Services is: (Specifically from the National Heart, Lung and Blood Institute: Obesity Education Initiative).

"*A diet that is individually planned to help create a deficit of 500 to 1,000 kcal/day should be an integral part of any program aimed at achieving a weight loss of 1 to 2 pounds per week.*"

What this is effectively telling you to do is to drive from John O'Groats to Lands End in the UK, or from the West to the East Coast of America, but without putting enough fuel in the car to do so ("*Eat less*"). Worse than that, you are then being told to flog the car even harder, so that it will conk out even sooner than it would have done, had you driven it to conserve energy ("*Do more*").

If a car mechanic seriously told you to do this to your car you would think they were mad and yet millions of people in the 'developed' world are deliberately trying to run their bodies on less fuel than they need, every single day.

This is the very idea of the calorie controlled diet – take in less fuel than you need. The theory is that your body will make up for the calorie deficit by burning fat that you have stored already, but it is not as simple as this. Your body first and foremost is a survival machine. The human body has developed over thousands of years and it has survived and adapted to far more challenging things than calorie counting.

We will see below exactly what your body will do when you try to follow this advice and it is pretty much the exact opposite of what you want it to do. At every stage it will do its best to 1) make you eat, 2) store fat and 3) conserve energy – all the things you **don't** want to happen.

Where does calorie counting come from?

Fact Box: The definition of a calorie is *"a unit of heat and energy equal to the amount of heat energy needed to raise the temperature of 1g of water by 1°C from 14.5°C to 15.5°C."*

In 1930, two American Doctors, (Newburgh & Johnson), wrote an article called *The Nature of Obesity*, which is generally seen as the first 'evidence' for the calorie theory. Newburgh & Johnson conclude *"Our evidence leads to the generalization that obesity is **always** caused by an inflow of energy that is greater than the outflow"* (my emphasis). If I tell you that this statement is based on little more than the observation of one of their lab staff for five days, you may understand Newburgh and Johnson's concern at how widely their work was adopted and my concern that this article still holds so much weight today.

An average male needs around 2500-3000 calories a day to live and an average female around 2000 calories a day. The calorie theory, as it has become known, says that if we eat 3500 calories fewer than we need, we will lose 1lb. So the theory tells us to deprive ourselves of 3500 calories for every pound we want to lose. This is where you get advice like *"cut your food intake by 500 calories a day and lose a pound a week"*. The theory here is that seven days worth of 500 fewer calories adds up to 3500 calories and that will be 1lb lost.

Does this calorie counting theory work?

The Calorie theory says – just eat 3500 fewer calories than your body needs and you will lose a pound. Full stop. No conditions are attached to this promise.

As we all know from our own experience, we can cut our calorie intake significantly and achieve results in the short term but, as time goes on, it becomes increasingly difficult to lose weight. The calorie theory doesn't allow for this – it simply says that if we have a deficit of 3500 calories we will lose a pound. The calorie theory, therefore, makes no distinction between the pounds lost at the start of a diet or the last few pounds to lose, to achieve our goal weight. We know that this is nonsense. We all know that the first seven pounds are so much easier to lose than the last.

If the calorie theory did work, I wouldn't be alive. I managed to survive for a year on fewer than 1000 calories a day – some days as little as 400 calories a day. If you do the maths, even assuming I never went below 1000 calories a day, this would still be at least 365 x 1000 calories fewer than I needed and this means I should have lost 104 pounds over the year – literally my entire body weight.

What did happen was that I lost weight quite rapidly to start with, but then my body adjusted to the food deprivation and adapted to having fewer calories. I lost lean muscle, stored fat and my metabolism slowed down dramatically. The weight loss slowed and then stopped and my body's ability to survive won through. I eventually got to the point where I would put on weight eating 1000 calories a day – I should still have been losing 2lb per week according to the calorie theory. The calorie theory may have some truth in the short term, but our body soon adjusts and we adapt to having fewer calories to ensure our survival. This then wrecks our chances of losing weight and keeping it off long term.

The simple and obvious answer to the question "*does this calorie counting theory work*?" is no! Not just because I am living proof that it doesn't work, but also because we have been giving this advice since the 1930's and we are just getting fatter and fatter as nations. We have been pushing this advice increasingly strongly since the 1980's and the numbers of obese and overweight people are going up, not down. Not only are they going up – they are galloping up at an astonishing rate. Could it be, therefore, that far from making the obesity epidemic better, this advice is actually making it worse? **This is my absolute belief. I am totally convinced that the calorie theory is the *cause* of the obesity epidemic, far from being the cure.**

For some more evidence, let us look at some direct quotes from the UK Food Standards Agency web site (taken from the site in 2007, so they may have been updated at the time you are reading this):

- *"The proportion of energy in our diets coming from fat is about the same as in the 1950s. In the 1960s and 1970s the energy from fat in our diets increased but since the late 1980s we have been consuming less total fat and we've also cut down on saturated fat"*;

- *"Since the 60s we've been consuming fewer calories from household food... However, there are an increasing number of people who are overweight or obese. The reasons for this are not clear..."*;

- *"Following significant changes over the past few years, the British diet is probably as healthy as it's ever been"*;

- *"Levels of obesity have tripled since 1980 in England, and there is no sign of the upward trend stopping"*;

- *"The UK has the fastest rising obesity rates in the developed world"*.

So, let me understand this, the UK has been following the diet advice – we are eating less fat, we are eating fewer calories, our diet is probably the best it has ever been, but levels of obesity have tripled since 1980 and we have the fastest rising obesity rate in the world. If this were a scientific experiment, you would stop it immediately and conclude that it isn't working. What happens instead is that the advice is shouted even louder and stronger by most governments, doctors and dieticians. *"Eat less, do more"* – that's the only advice they can give us.

If only it were that simple, we wouldn't have an obesity problem, let alone an epidemic. I firmly believe that the calorie theory will go down as one of the most serious myths in history. Just as we came to realise how bad smoking is for people's health, so I believe that we will come to realise that telling people to "*eat less, do more*" has **caused** our current obesity crisis. Far from it ever being the cure, I think that it is the **cause**.

The reason that this advice makes the obesity problem worse, is because of what happens to us when we try to eat less and do more...

What happens DIRECTLY when we count calories?

There are three direct things that happen when we try to eat less energy than our body needs:

1) We get hungry;

2) Our bodies store fat and use up lean muscle;

3) Our metabolisms slow down, to conserve the limited energy that we have, and this means we need fewer calories to live on.

Let's look at each of these, for a quick and simple explanation:

1) The first thing that happens, when we try to eat less, is that we get hungry. As soon as you eat less than your body needs, your body sends out signals to try to get you to eat. Your body doesn't know that you have read a diet book. It thinks you have landed on a desert island and have been forced into a life threatening starvation situation and it tries to look after you.

You will be very familiar with the signals that your body sends out to try to get you to eat. Physical symptoms include: shaky hands; sweaty palms; feeling light headed; headaches and a rumbly tummy are some of the best examples.

Mental/emotional symptoms include: irritability; inability to concentrate; indecisiveness and an unusually high preoccupation with food. It is no coincidence that, as soon as you start a calorie-controlled diet, all you can think about is food. This is your body telling you to eat.

The first fact – your body making you hungry – is enough to ruin most diets. You start a new diet with such good intentions, but you are trying to fight your body from the start and your body will always win. (You're going to learn in this book how to start working **with** your body to lose weight and it is far easier and more effective – trust me).

2) The second thing that happens, when you try to eat less than you need, is that your body stores fat and uses up lean muscle. This is the exact opposite of what you want to happen. You want to get rid of the fat and keep the lean muscle, but your body won't do this and here is why. Lean muscle uses up more calories (energy) than fat does. Back to the desert island situation – your body is in survival mode when you try to eat less, so it needs to 'dump' the part of you that needs the most energy. This is the lean muscle – so that needs to go first. Your body hangs on to the fat a) because it uses up less energy and b) because it is going to be a valuable reserve if you are on the 'desert island' for a long time.

This is a double whammy for you a) because you want to lose fat, not nice, toned, lean muscle and b) because the more lean muscle you have, the higher your metabolism is. So, if you lose lean muscle, you reduce the number of calories that you can eat without putting on weight.

3) The third thing that happens, when you try to eat less than you need, is that your metabolism slows down. Your body does this to conserve the limited

energy that is now coming in. This then means, as with (2) above, you will need fewer calories to live on and you will put on weight if you try to eat the number of calories that used to maintain your weight.

What happens INDIRECTLY when we count calories?

If the direct things that happen, when you try to eat less than you need, haven't totally put you off counting calories, let's go a bit further. The completely new and key impact of this book is the next bit. The research I have done shows that there are three medical conditions that cause insatiable food cravings.

These three conditions are Candida, Food Intolerance and Hypoglycaemia. They have been known about and written about for years – over 100 years, in the case of Hypoglycaemia. If you can't stick to a diet and you have cravings for things like biscuits, cakes, chocolate, cereal and even fruit, I would put money on you having one, two, or all three of these conditions. If you have one of the conditions, the chances are you have two or three of them, because they are so inter-connected. So your body could have all three conditions causing you to crave certain foods.

Doctors and authors who have written about these conditions have talked, almost in passing, about the impact that they have on weight and food cravings. They haven't put all the evidence together and discovered why people can't stick to a diet. This book has and, in so doing, two unique contributions of this book are to show:

- That these three conditions cause unbelievable food cravings and

- That Calorie counting is almost guaranteed to cause these conditions.

In short, therefore, if you follow the current diet advice – "*eat less, do more*" – you are extremely likely to develop the three conditions that cause food cravings. So, start a calorie-controlled diet and end up a food addict. It really is as scary as that.

Let's see now how calorie counting can lead to these three conditions. We need another fact box, just before we do this, to make sure we know the basics about food – carbohydrate, protein and fat.

Fact Box: All food is carbohydrate, protein or fat – or a combination of two or three of those. Fruit is mostly carbohydrate, with some protein and virtually no fat. Meat is protein and fat and has no carbohydrate. Forget protein, as protein is in everything from lettuce to bread to fish. The two really interesting food groups are carbohydrates and fats. Both have protein in them, so, I'll say it again – don't worry about protein.

The best way to remember the difference between a carbohydrate and a fat is that a fat either had a face, or comes from something with a face. All meat and fish were animals – with faces. Eggs, butter and cheese all come from animals – with faces. The exceptions are healthy oils like sunflower oil and olive oil (which come from sunflowers and olives), but don't worry about these – the only fats you need to think about are the ones from the faces.

When we start a calorie-controlled diet we do the following:

1) We increase the proportion of carbohydrates in our diet;

2) We reduce the variety of food eaten;

3) We weaken our immune systems.

We're now going to understand why trying to eat less is going to lead to 1) 2) and 3) above and why these three things then cause Candida, Food Intolerance and Hypoglycaemia.

1) If you count calories you will increase the proportion of carbohydrates in your diet. Quite simply, gram for gram, carbs are always lower in calories than fat. Fat has approximately nine calories per gram while carbohydrate has four. If you know this, when you are trying to cut back on calories, you will avoid fat and choose carbohydrates instead – as the lower calorie option. Even if you don't know this, you may know the calorie content of certain foods and you may know that you could have half a dozen apples for the calorie equivalent of a salmon fillet. As the carbohydrate options are always lower in calories than fat options, gram for gram, calorie counters tend to increase the proportion of carbohydrates in their diet and reduce the proportion of fat.

If you don't do your own calorie counting, but you follow a diet from a magazine, or any low fat/calorie controlled book, the diet will automatically do the calorie counting for you. Sometimes the diet will tell you how many calories a day you will be having. Weight Watchers ® has a points system – this is calorie counting 'made easy'. Some low fat diets don't spell out the calorie count for you, but they recommend carbohydrate options for you, to make sure that you avoid fat. On any low calorie/low fat diet, your basic diet foods will be fruit, crisp breads, salads, cereal bars, maybe cereal like *"Special K"*® – all carbohydrates. Steak, oily fish, cheese, milk, olive oil and other fats will barely get a mention in any calorie-controlled diet.

All the advice that we have had for decades, on eating lower fat foods, just ensures that we have more carbohydrate in our diets. Since everything is mainly a carbohydrate food or a fat food, avoiding fats means that you increase the proportion of carbohydrates in your diet. This is simply a mathematical fact.

So, counting calories/trying to eat less/following a low fat diet – are all based on the calorie theory in one way or another and they all lead to an increase in the proportion of carbohydrates in your diet. We will also see in the next few pages how carbohydrates lead to the three medical conditions – Candida, Food Intolerance and Hypoglycaemia.

2) The second thing that we do, when we start a calorie-controlled diet, is to reduce the variety of foods eaten. We tend to go for the regular favourites that give us 'the biggest bang for the buck' (the most food for the fewest calories). We probably have a set breakfast – our calorie counted bread, or cereal, every day. We probably have a set lunch also – a shop bought calorie-counted ready meal or calorie counted sandwich or cereal bar. We may vary the evening meal a bit more, but it is still likely to have the same ingredients in it and always more carbs than fats.

Hold this thought and again, we will see, in the next few pages, the problem with eating a limited variety of foods for the three medical conditions – Candida, Food Intolerance and Hypoglycaemia.

3) The third thing that we do when we count calories is weaken our immune systems. This happens in the following ways:

a) Simply because we are not eating as much fuel as our bodies need, we are denying our bodies much needed energy;

b) On top of this we have just seen that we eat more carbohydrates and cut back on fats. Fats are essential for our wellbeing because they form the membrane (thin protection layer) that surrounds every cell in our bodies;

c) We also develop nutritional deficiencies when we don't eat enough, because we don't get enough fats, calories and we eat a limited variety of foods.

In Part 3 of this book, we will go into all the basic details about the three conditions – What is, say, Candida? What causes it? How do we know if we've got it? How does it cause food cravings/addiction? How do we get rid of it?

At this stage of the book, it is just important to know that 1) eating more carbohydrates, 2) having a limited variety of foods and 3) weakening our immune systems all lead to the three conditions that cause food cravings:

1) Increasing the proportion of carbohydrates in our diet is bad for all three conditions:

   - Candida thrives on carbohydrates, whilst fats have no impact on it at all (some fats even kill it off);

   - The most common Food Intolerances are to carbohydrates – wheat, sugar and corn. Intolerance to meat, fish or oils is almost unheard of;

   - Finally, Hypoglycaemia is directly related to carbohydrates. Remember, Hypoglycaemia is a word to describe the state your body is in if your blood glucose level is too low. Only carbohydrates affect your blood glucose level. Pure fats don't have any harmful effect at all.

2) Reducing the variety of food eaten is again bad for all three conditions, especially when the limited foods eaten are generally carbohydrates:

- Eating dieters' staple foods of low calorie cereal, low calorie bread, calorie counted processed meals, fruit and sweet 'treats' feeds Candida beautifully;

- The very definition of Food Intolerance is eating the same food too much, too often. So reducing the variety of foods eaten has a clear and direct impact on Food Intolerance;

- With Hypoglycaemia – eating the same carbohydrates regularly continues to have bad effects on our blood glucose levels.

3) Weakening our immune systems, by not eating enough calories and by not eating enough fat, makes our bodies more likely to get all three of the conditions. A weakened immune system leads to:

- Candida, as it creates the environment for the yeast to multiply;

- Food Intolerance, as our bodies are more susceptible to adverse reactions to common foods;

- Hypoglycaemia, as our general health is likely to impact our blood glucose level and stability.

In summary, counting calories will make you eat more carbohydrates (relative to fats). It will reduce the variety of foods that you eat and it will weaken your immune system. These, in turn, all lay your body wide open to Candida, Food Intolerance and Hypoglycaemia. Get these and you will crave foods (carbohydrates mainly) like an addict.

So, start counting calories and settle down to a life of uncontrollable cravings and food obsession. Stop counting calories and start losing weight!

Stop counting calories & start losing weight

Hopefully by now you realise that, as soon as you try to eat less, let alone do more, you are going to **directly** make your body work against you and you are **indirectly** going to do things that give you some pretty nasty medical conditions, which will make you crave food.

Directly the following will happen:

1) You will get hungry;

2) Your body will store fat and use up lean muscle;

3) Your metabolism will slow down, to conserve the limited energy that you have, and this means you need fewer calories to live on.

Indirectly the following will happen:

1) You will increase the proportion of carbohydrates in your diet;

2) You will reduce the variety of food eaten;

3) You will weaken your immune systems.

You will then, most likely, develop Candida, Food Intolerance and/or Hypoglycaemia and the food cravings that go with all these. To lose weight you have to stop food cravings, so that you can stick to a healthy diet. To stop food cravings you have to eat enough, so that you're not hungry, and get rid of these three conditions and stop them coming back. You have to "**Stop counting calories, therefore, to start losing weight.**"

I know that this may contradict everything that you have been told over many years, but it is so important that you accept that counting calories does not work, in the long run, before moving on. It will take a transformation of your previous thinking habits to be successful from now on in the dieting war.

For years you have been taught to count calories and reduce your calorie intake below what you should eat for health and energy. You have gone hungry, you have viewed fat as the devil. You have eaten bland, tasteless foods. You have felt deprived. You have probably had some success, only to put weight back on. Or you are a relatively slim person at the moment, but you are reading this book to escape the constant battle of bingeing and starving. Or you may be at the point where you just cannot face depriving yourself one more day.

It is going to take some people quite a lot of time to stop eating less. Women particularly, have been in a state of controlled eating and abstinence for so long that it is very difficult for them to start eating well again.

The bottom line is that you wouldn't be reading this book if calorie counting did work. We have all tried low calorie diets and we now find we can no longer lose weight. It is a frequently documented fact that 95% of people who have lost weight on a low calorie diet put it back on within months and often more than they originally lost. Some research has estimated this figure to be as high as 98%. If it really were as simple as "*eat less than your body needs and you will lose weight*", we would have managed it years ago.

I have worked with so many people who couldn't let go of counting calories when they started The Harcombe Diet. They felt that if they didn't count calories they would overeat and gain weight. In fact they found the exact opposite. They ate more, lost the cravings and gained control over their eating in a way they never imagined possible. You can too...

Don't hang onto a lie that has not served you well in the past and has made you fatter and less able to lose weight today. The definition of madness is doing the same thing again and again and expecting a different result. You have to try something different, so keep reading and keep that mind open.

1) The first thing that you have to do is to stop calorie counting/eating less. Before you panic and throw this book away, ask yourself why you are reading it. Has calorie counting worked for you? Have you lost weight and kept it off? Are you at your ideal weight and are you free from food cravings? No!

Calorie counting has got you into the mess you're in now and stopping it is the only way out. Not only does calorie counting not work, it leads directly and indirectly to food cravings, which is the reason why you overeat. You have to stop counting calories if you want to lose weight. Have faith, dare to try something different and please keep reading.

2) The second thing that you have to do is to understand which of the three conditions you are suffering from, identify the foods that contribute to these conditions and stop eating these foods. You don't go 'cold turkey' on food but you do go 'cold turkey' on the foods that are contributing to your addict-like cravings. There are bad foods. Some food is good for you and some is not and you have to start nourishing your body, not stuffing and starving it. You also have to stop trying to be an addict in moderation. You are trying to stop being a smoker by having a few a day. You are trying to stop being an alcoholic by having a couple of glasses a day. Eating what you crave in moderation really is that crazy.

You are not weak-willed. It is not your fault that you are overweight or that you overeat. You are up against some physical cravings that are quite overwhelming. Take the first step to fighting them and read this book. It will help you achieve all of the above and more. More energy, better health and a life free from food addiction.

Part 3
The Medical Conditions

3
Candida

What is Candida?

Candida's full name is Candida Albicans, but we'll just call it Candida from now on. Candida is a yeast that lives in all of us. It is normally kept under control by our immune system and by other 'good' bacteria in our body. It usually lives in our digestive system. Women know they have an overgrowth of Candida when they get thrush. This is often called "*a yeast infection*". Athlete's foot and dandruff, as other examples, are generally signs of yeast infections/Candida.

Candida serves no useful purpose in your body (unlike other 'good' bacteria such as lactobacillus acidophilus). Provided it stays under control, you won't really know it is there and it doesn't cause any problems. In many people this yeast causes no harm and lives within them peacefully. The problem starts when Candida gets out of control and it can lead to all sorts of nasty symptoms.

Yeast exists just about everywhere on earth, living off other living things. In the right environment, yeast can reproduce at an alarming rate, as anyone who has ever made bread, wine or beer will know. Science has shown that a single yeast cell, given the right reproductive environment, can multiply to over one hundred yeast cells within twenty-four hours. In the human body, therefore, given the right environment, this normally harmless yeast can multiply to frightening levels and cause significant impact on our health and wellbeing.

What causes Candida overgrowth?

Or put another way – if yeast can multiply to frightening levels given the right environment – what makes our body the right environment for Candida to multiply?

There are five key things that turn our bodies into a perfect environment for Candida to get out of control:

1) A weakened immune system;

2) Eating things that feed Candida;

3) Medication – steroids, antibiotics, birth control pills, hormones;

4) Diabetes;

5) Nutritional deficiency.

1) A weakened immune system – If you have a weakened immune system you are more susceptible to Candida overgrowth and in fact Candida overgrowth is often seen as evidence of a weakened immune system. One will make the other worse in a vicious circle. If you have had a period of illness, or significant personal or work stress, the chances are that your immune system will be weaker than normal and this provides an ideal opportunity for Candida to multiply. This will then further weaken your immune system, as the Candida takes over and makes you feel awful.

2) Eating things that feed Candida – Anyone who has made beer at home will know the effect of mixing yeast, sugar and vinegar. The effect on Candida is much the same. The yeast thrives on all carbohydrates (especially processed ones), concentrated fruit sugar, yeast and vinegary/pickled foods. The fact that Candida became a significant health issue in the twentieth century is not surprising given the recent increase in processed food consumption. As we have increased our consumption of processed foods, we have fed the

parasite Candida in our body and enabled it to get out of balance.

3) Medication – There are many modern medicines that upset our natural body harmony and encourage the overgrowth of Candida. These include steroids, antibiotics, birth control pills and hormones, all of which were unknown before the twentieth century. This is another reason why Candida and the related obesity problems have become far more wide-spread in recent years. Antibiotics, and other modern medicines, kill off the good bacteria in our intestines – like lactobacilli. Lactobacilli are part of the 'friendly' gut bacteria that keep Candida under control. So, when we take antibiotics, steroids or the pill, we kill off the good bacteria and allow Candida to get out of control.

4) Diabetes – when we eat a carbohydrate, our body produces insulin to get our blood glucose level back to normal. In a Diabetic this doesn't happen, because the organ that makes insulin (the pancreas) doesn't work. This is what it means to be diabetic.

Diabetes is sometimes called *"sweet urine"* and doctors test for Diabetes by asking you to give a urine sample and then seeing if there is sugar in your sample. This 'sweet' body environment, which Diabetics have, is a great breeding ground for Candida. It is well-known that Diabetics struggle more with their weight than the average non-Diabetic and there could be a few reasons for this:

- The injections of insulin lead directly to weight problems, as insulin is the fattening hormone;

- Diabetics are more prone to Candida with their sugary body environment and, therefore, the cravings linked to Candida are likely to be making them fat;

- Diabetics don't have a natural mechanism to regulate their blood glucose level and are, therefore, trying to balance injections with food consumed at all times. They are, therefore, likely to get food cravings if this balance is out of sync at any time.

5) Nutritional Deficiency – There is much evidence to suggest that our nutritional deficiency has actually got worse and not better as we have 'developed' as nations. Analysis in the UK reveals that the war time diet, when food was rationed, was actually better for us than our current diet, where we can freely choose from every food available. In war time we were limited to fixed amounts of meat, fish, vegetables, fruits, dairy products and grains, but we were also limited in our access to sugar and other processed foods. In comparison with current diets, high in processed foods, our predecessors ate quite well. We may be overeating as developed nations but we are certainly not over consuming vitamins. A number of nutrients are key to the control of Candida and there is evidence that they are lacking in our current diets:

- Biotin, one of the B vitamins, can help prevent the conversion of the yeast form of Candida to its fungal form. One of the richest sources of Biotin is pigs' kidneys while reasonable sources are eggs and whole grains. How often do you eat these?

- Vitamin C affects general immunity, which impacts the environment in which yeast can multiply. Stress also destroys vitamin C and we may not be getting the levels of Vitamin C we need for optimal health and immunity with our current 'fast food' diets. The body does not store Vitamin C, so we need a constant supply to keep Candida at bay.

- B vitamins are also needed for stress tolerance and the immune system and we lose valuable sources of B vitamins when we choose processed carbohydrates over wholemeal carbohydrates. Cereals and breads are often fortified with added vitamins and these are the only sources of B vitamins in many of our diets. However, these come in products laden with sugar and other processed carbohydrates so we would be better off avoiding them altogether and eating the whole foods, or taking a vitamin pill on its own.

- Magnesium, selenium and zinc are the key minerals needed for the immune system and we generally find that modern diets are lacking in all three of these. Magnesium is found in Soya beans, nuts and whole grains. Selenium is found in kidneys and liver, fish and shellfish and whole grains. Zinc is found in oysters, meat, fish and shellfish and hard cheese. If your diet is lacking in nuts, whole grains, high quality fish, shellfish and meat you may well be lacking in any, or all, of these minerals.

All of the nutritional deficiencies highlighted above can create the environment in which Candida can multiply within us.

How do you know if you have Candida overgrowth?

In general, chronic Candida overgrowth can make a person feel very unwell all over. Here are some of the many symptoms that you may be experiencing if you have Candida overgrowth:

Stomach – constipation; diarrhoea; irritable bowel syndrome; bloating, especially after eating; two sets of clothes needed for pre and post eating; indigestion; gas; heartburn.

Head – headaches; dizziness; blurred vision; flushed cheeks; feeling of 'sleepwalking'; feeling unreal; feeling 'spaced out'.

Women – Pre-Menstrual Tension (PMT); water retention; irregular periods; vaginal discharge or itchiness; thrush; cystitis.

Blood Glucose – hungry between meals; irritable or moody before meals; feeling faint/shaky when food is not eaten; irregular pulse before and after eating; headaches late morning and late afternoon; waking in the early hours and not being able to get back to sleep; abnormal cravings for sweet foods/bread/ alcohol or caffeine; eating sweets makes you more hungry; excessive appetite; instant sugar 'high' followed by fatigue; chilly feeling after eating.

Mental – anxiety; depression; irritability; lethargy; memory problems; loss of concentration; moodiness; nightmares; mental 'sluggishness'; *"get up and go"* has got up and gone.

Other – dramatic fluctuations in weight from one day to the next; easy weight gain; poor circulation; hands and feet sensitive to cold; feeling of being unable to cope; constant fatigue; muscle aches or cramps; sighing often – 'hunger for air'; yawning easily; difficulty sleeping; excessive thirst; coated tongue; dry skin; hair loss; symptoms worse after consuming yeast or sugary foods; symptoms worse on damp, humid or rainy days; athletes foot; dandruff or other fungal infections.

As you can see, the complaints linked to Candida are many and varied. If you are feeling very unwell at the moment you may identify with many of the above symptoms and you may be as worried about your general health as you are about your eating habits. However, many readers will be most aware of the sugar handling problems, water retention, fatigue, easy weight gain, dramatic fluctuations in weight, stomach bloating, depression, anxiety and other symptoms common to eating problems. If Candida is left unchecked you could soon develop many of the other symptoms until your health deteriorates to an unprecedented level. Candida does not get better on its own – it gets worse. At the moment you may just be worried about sugar cravings and weight fluctuations, but things could get a lot worse.

If you need a check list to add to the above, the following questionnaire should help you identify if Candida is a problem for you. The questionnaire on the next page shows the **causes** of Candida. If you have many of the things that can cause Candida you may well find that this is a problem for you.

Questionnaire 1 – Causes

	YES's
Immune System:	
- Have you been 'off sick' in the last 2 years?	
'Feeding' Candida:	
- Do you eat processed foods at least once a day? (Sugar, white flour, white rice, white pasta, cakes, biscuits, confectionery etc)	
- Do you eat more portions of carbohydrates (including fruit) than fat each day?	
Medication:	
- Do you remember taking antibiotics during childhood?	
- Have you taken antibiotics during adulthood?	
- Have you been on 'the pill'?	
- Have you taken hormones in any other form?	
- Have you ever taken steroids? (e.g. predisone or cortisone)	
- Have you ever been pregnant?	
Diabetes:	
- Are you Diabetic?	
Nutritional Deficiency:	
Do you have any signs of nutritional deficiency?	
- White spots on finger nails,	
- Dry flaky skin or brittle hair or nails,	
- Poor hair or skin condition,	
- Muscle aches or general tiredness,	
- Dull, dry eyes	

The more times you answered 'yes' and the more sections out of the five that had at least one 'yes'; the more likely you are to have Candida, as you will be showing strong evidence for the causes of Candida. If you answer 'Yes' in each of the five sections you have been exposed to all the key causes of Candida and, therefore, you will almost certainly be suffering from this condition. You can still be a sufferer answering 'yes' in just one or two of the sections.

Having looked at the **causes**, we move onto the **symptoms**. The following questionnaire looks at the symptoms of Candida and whether or not you have an overgrowth of Candida.

In the following table please score as follows:

- 1 point for each symptom that is occasional and mild;

- 2 points for each symptom that is frequent and moderate/quite strong;

- 3 points for each symptom that is continuous and significant/very strong.

Questionnaire 2 – Symptoms

	POINTS
Stomach: (Maximum 21) - Constipation - Diarrhoea - Irritable bowel syndrome - Bloating, especially after eating - Indigestion - Gas - Heartburn	
Head: (Maximum 21) - Headaches - Dizziness - Blurred vision - Flushed cheeks - Feeling of 'sleepwalking' - Feeling unreal - Feeling 'spaced out'	
Women: (Maximum 18) - PMT - Water retention - Irregular periods - Vaginal discharge or itchiness - Thrush - Cystitis	

<u>Blood Glucose</u>: (Maximum 30) - Hungry between meals - Irritable or moody before meals - Feeling faint/shaky when food is not eaten - Headaches late morning and late afternoon - Waking in the early hours and not being able to get back to sleep - Abnormal cravings for sweet foods, bread, alcohol or caffeine - Eating sweets makes you more hungry - Excessive appetite - Instant sugar 'high' followed by fatigue - Chilly feeling after eating	
<u>Mental</u>: (Maximum 30) - Anxiety - Depression - Irritability - Lethargy - Memory problems - Loss of concentration - Moodiness - Nightmares - Mental 'sluggishness' - *"Get up and go"* has got up and gone	
<u>Other</u> : (Maximum 51) - Dramatic fluctuations in weight from one day to the next	

- Easy weight gain	
- Poor circulation	
- Hands and feet sensitive to cold	
- Feeling of being unable to cope	
- Constant fatigue	
- Muscle aches or cramps	
- Sighing often – 'hunger for air'	
- Yawning easily	
- Difficulty sleeping	
- Excessive thirst	
- Coated tongue	
- Dry skin	
- Hair loss	
- Symptoms worse after consuming yeasty or sugary foods	
- Symptoms worse on damp, humid or rainy days	
- Athletes foot, dandruff or other fungal infection	

Again – the more points scored, and the more sections the points were scored in, the more likely it is that Candida is a problem for you. If you scored more than 50 points, and scored in three or more sections, it is very likely that you are suffering from Candida.

Please note that both these questionnaires are on *www.theharcombediet.com* – so you can print them off and re-do them any time you like.

How does Candida cause food cravings?

Candida is a living organism and every living thing has a natural self-preservation mechanism – we all fight to survive. The yeast living inside us is exactly the same. The Candida needs carbohydrates, especially processed carbohydrates, to feed it. It thrives on a weak immune system. It hates garlic and nutrients, as they attack it and kill it off.

If you have Candida, you are having a constant battle with your body – you are trying to feel well but the Candida is trying to survive. The things needed for your wellbeing and the Candida's wellbeing are the opposite. When Candida really takes hold you will crave the foods that feed the yeast to ensure it grows and flourishes. If you crave burgers, you may well be craving the ketchup you put on them or the sugar, breadcrumbs and preservatives added to the meat. If you crave salad, it may well be the dressing that you are really after, with its vinegar and sugar ingredients. You can pretty much guarantee you are not craving naked lettuce leaves and plain grilled meat.

You crave the things that feed the yeast, therefore, – all sugary foods, processed foods, concentrated fruit sugar, yeast and yeast derivatives and vinegary/pickled foods. There is evidence to suggest that eating yeast itself does not feed the yeast, but the consumption of bread and other foods containing yeast generally maintains the environment that the yeast needs to thrive in your body.

There are case studies throughout books on Candida, which give specific examples of the food cravings experienced by Candida sufferers. There are many other references in magazine articles, web pages and books on Candida. It is an absolutely documented fact that people with Candida overgrowth experience addict-like food cravings. People will drive to a grocery store in the middle of the night to feed the cravings and in so doing they will feed the yeast driving the cravings and make the cravings even worse in the future. The more you give into the cravings, the worse the Candida will get and the worse the cravings will get. It really is a vicious circle.

The good news is that there is a virtuous circle, which is just as easy to get into, if you can break the vicious circle. The virtuous circle goes something like – you don't give into the cravings, you fight the yeast with diet and supplements, the cravings get easier, you get stronger, the Candida gets weaker, the cravings get easier and so on. The more you give into Candida fed cravings the worse they will get – you have to break the cycle and free yourself from the cravings that are ruining your desire to be slim and probably your overall health and life.

How can you treat Candida?

There are some excellent writers who have focused on Candida such as Leon Chaitow, John Parks Trowbridge & Morton Walker and William G. Crook. There are three main pieces of advice for people suffering from Candida:

1) Starve the Candida overgrowth with diet;

2) Attack the Candida overgrowth with supplements that kill the yeast;

3) Treat the causes so that it doesn't come back.

1) **Starve the Candida**. The first thing we must do is to stop feeding the Candida – this means no processed foods, no sugary foods, no vinegary foods and even good carbohydrates, like fruit and whole-grains, must be restricted for a while. What you can eat is best summed up by Trowbridge & Walker's quite memorable expression "MEVY" – **M**eat/fish, **E**ggs, **V**egetables and **Y**oghurt (NLY – Natural Live Yoghurt).

2) **Attack the Candida** overgrowth with supplements that kill the yeast. Candida hates all of the following:

- Garlic – scientists have shown that garlic added to colonies of bacteria have stopped the functioning of that bacteria in minutes. Hence garlic is a well-known and well-documented antibacterial agent. Garlic has also been shown to be an effective weapon against yeast and fungi;

- Biotin – research has shown that where a Biotin deficiency exists, Candida changes more rapidly from its relatively harmless yeast form to its more dangerous multiplying form. So Biotin has been shown to be a most useful vitamin in controlling Candida overgrowth;

- Olive oil – contains oleic acid, which stops the growth of the yeast in much the same way as Biotin;

- Caprylic acid – which comes from coconut oil. You can get user friendly versions of this from some health food shops or from Internet suppliers;

- Lactobacillus Acidophilus – this is one of the major 'friendly' bacteria in our digestive systems and it can, therefore, be used to re-balance the gut flora and to fight off the Candida. Again health food shops and Internet suppliers will have this.

3) **Treat the cause** so that it doesn't return. Go back to the 'What causes Candida overgrowth?' section and see where the roots for your problem were:

- A weakened immune system – eat well, drink plenty of water, don't smoke, drink alcohol in moderation, take time out to do things you enjoy, laugh, socialise, strive for balance. We all know the many things we can do to keep our health optimal and our immune system the strongest it can be;

- Eating things that feed Candida – don't go back to consuming lots of sugary, yeasty, vinegary foods once you have got Candida back under control, or you will be asking for it to return;

- Medication – steroids, antibiotics, birth control pills, hormones – try to avoid taking any of these if at all possible. Clearly serious illness requires treatment and unwanted pregnancies are not to be risked, but try to avoid taking any of the above if you can. Is there an alternative form of contraception? See if you can heal a mild infection with Vitamin C and natural remedies before reaching for the antibiotics etc;

- Diabetes – you can still do things to help your situation if Diabetes is the cause of your yeast overgrowth. You can eat as healthy a diet as possible and thereby reduce the level of glucose in your blood, which may cause yeast overgrowth. Some individuals have been able to reduce the level of insulin they take and some even come off it altogether by following diets with little or no carbohydrates. If you are insulin dependent you must work with your doctor to work out the best diet and level of insulin for you. One thing that you can be sure of is that your health can only improve with the elimination of processed foods from your diet;

- Nutritional deficiency – eat as wide a variety as possible of vegetables, protein, whole grains, pulses and fruits and you should have no problem with nutritional deficiency. The most common causes of nutritional deficiency in the developed world are self inflicted – smoking, drinking too much alcohol, dieting and eating processed foods, leaving little room for more nutritious foods.

Top tips for motivation

This is about as horrible as common medical conditions go. There is a parasite inside you, which is demanding to be fed, leading to you feeling dreadful – overweight, spaced out, tired, bloated and hardly able to get through the day. This parasite thrives on sugar, vinegary foods and yeast, as anyone who makes beer or wine will know. The more you feed it, the stronger it gets and the weaker you get.

This is war! Don't give this parasite anything it wants. Starve it by depriving it of all the foods it wants and kill it with supplements that it hates. How dare this thing try to take over your body? The good news is that you can devastate it very quickly in the battle. After just five days on a strict anti-Candida diet (Phase 1) you can do a whole heap of damage. You may have cravings like you have never known, in the early stages, and you could experience some quite unpleasant 'die-off' symptoms, as you kill the yeast, but this should only serve to strengthen your resolve. You may feel temporarily worse but soon you will start feeling quite dramatically better. Even after these first five tough days you could be feeling more energetic, less spaced out, the cravings should have subsided substantially and you will have lost pounds in weight.

Just imagine that every time you put a processed carbohydrate or vinegary food in your mouth you are putting petrol into the Candida's tank – you are literally fuelling this parasite that is making your life a misery. Keep this image in your mind every time you have a craving and you will soon rather do anything than feed this monster. Don't see processed carbohydrates as delicious – they are petrol for the enemy. Just visualise bacteria multiplying in your body with every mouthful you eat and this should ease the cravings.

If you don't attack this parasite it will just get stronger and stronger and you will feel weaker and weaker. You have to get it back in control sometime so start straight away before it gets any worse. Think of an end to tiredness and cravings. Think of an end to stomach bloating and digestive problems. Think of this horrible thing in your body and go for it.

Quick Summary on Candida

• Candida is a yeast that lives in all of us. It serves no useful purpose. When it gets out of control it can create havoc in our bodies.

• The main causes of Candida are 1) a weakened immune system, 2) eating things that feed Candida, 3) medication, such as antibiotics and steroids, 4) Diabetes and 5) nutritional deficiency.

• A wide variety of symptoms – physical and psychological – can indicate that Candida is overgrown inside you.

• Candida contributes to food cravings by demanding that you feed it – it loves processed carbohydrates, yeast and sugar in particular. This parasite can produce uncontrollable food cravings as it drives you to feed it so it can grow more and produce even stronger food cravings.

• You can treat it with a three step approach – 1) starve the Candida with your diet 2) attack the Candida overgrowth with supplements like garlic and 3) treat the causes so that it doesn't come back.

• This is war! You have to kill off this parasite before it does any more harm inside your body.

4

Food Intolerance

What is Food Intolerance?

The dictionary definition of 'allergy' is:

"The condition of reacting adversely to certain substances – especially food or pollen."

Just to be clear, in this chapter, we are talking about Food Intolerance and not allergy, as defined above. Food allergy refers to potentially fatal reactions to a substance, such as with nut allergies. If someone has a food allergy the chances are that they were born with this allergy, will always have this allergy and it is a very serious condition.

Common allergenic foods include nuts, shellfish, strawberries, I even know someone violently allergic to kiwis. If a person is exposed to the food, to which they are allergic, reactions range from breaking out into a rash, to extreme vomiting/stomach upset, or even death. We have all read tragic cases where people with an extreme allergy have died from being exposed to the food to which they are allergic. The sensitivity is extraordinary – my cousin discovered her young child had a nut allergy when she kissed him on the cheek, hours after she had eaten a Chinese meal that contained peanut oil. Her son reacted to the tiny trace of oil in the kiss on his cheek.

This chapter is not about **food allergy**. It is about **Food Intolerance**, which literally means having an intolerance to a particular food or foods. By intolerance we mean an adverse reaction – not an extreme life threatening reaction as with food allergy – but any adverse reaction, which causes the person discomfort. Adverse reactions can include anything from gastrointestinal disorders to headaches and reactions

M _Hope_

HAS AN APPOINTMENT ON

☐ MON. ☐ TUES. ☐ WED. ☐ THURS. ☐ FRI. ☐ SAT.

DATE 6/10/10 AT 10:45 ☐ A.M. ☐ P.M.

J.M. GILMORE, M.D.
BOARD CERTIFIED ENDOCRINOLOGIST

725 RESERVOIR AVENUE

(401) 943-5120   CRANSTON, R.I. 02910

IF UNABLE TO KEEP APPOINTMENT, KINDLY GIVE ONE FULL BUSINESS DAY NOTICE

that affect the mental state of the person who has consumed the food.

What causes Food Intolerance?

Food Intolerance develops with repeated overexposure to a particular food. The key words here are 'repeated' and 'overexposure'. It is common for people to become intolerant to foods that they eat a lot of and on a regular basis.

The foods most likely to cause intolerance are, therefore, the ones that are consumed most of and most often. The most common foods in the US to cause sensitivity are:

1) Dairy products

2) Wheat

3) Corn *

4) Eggs

5) Soy *

6) Peanuts *

7) Sugar

    * Corn, Soy and Peanuts are eaten very frequently in the US but far less so in the UK.

In Australia, the most common Food Intolerances are to milk and wheat. Dr Brostoff, one of the leading Food Intolerance specialists in the UK, lists the most common foods causing intolerance in the UK also as milk and wheat. Dr Brostoff also noted that for a doctor working in Taiwan, rice and soya beans were the chief culprits. The finger should point at whichever foods are most commonly eaten in the local cuisine.

It is estimated that we rely on as few as a dozen foods on a daily basis and that almost all of these will come from the milk, sugar and wheat food families. We eat toast or cereal for breakfast with milk (milk, sugar and wheat). We often have sugary snacks, and milk in tea and coffee, throughout the day (milk, sugar and wheat). We may have pasta, sandwiches or pizza for main meals (wheat and often milk and sugar again). If we have a salad, meat or fish, we may well have wheat or dairy with it, such as cheese, bread or crisp breads and so on. (You may like to count how many different basic substances – like wheat – you eat on a regular basis and it may not even exceed 20).

With repeated overexposure to any food, our bodies can become intolerant to this food and we will start to experience withdrawal symptoms if we don't have the food (this is when we are officially addicted to the food and the cravings for the food will be making us overeat).

There are other things that happen to make us more susceptible to Food Intolerance. Illness and medication can lead to a weakened immune system that will make us more susceptible to Food Intolerance and then this in turn weakens our immune system further (we are in a vicious circle downwards at this stage). Counting calories can also lead to Food Intolerance, as we saw in Part 2, for a couple of reasons:

- We can weaken our immune system by taking in less fuel than we need.

- We tend to eat a restricted variety of foods when we count calories – we tend to eat more fruit and other low calorie foods and cut out steak, dairy products and other high calorie foods. As we restrict the variety of foods that we eat, sticking to our favourites that fill us up as much as possible for as few calories as possible, we are starting down the slippery slope towards Food Intolerance.

Food Allergies are invariably constant throughout life, but Food Intolerance is not fixed and it can vary over time. People can find themselves susceptible to certain foods at different stages of their lives. For example, someone suffering from stress can develop intolerance to a food that they are consuming a lot of at that time and then be able to eat the food again in moderation at other times in their life. Pregnant women sometimes develop a sensitivity to a particular food that disappears after childbirth. My mother, for example, developed a sensitivity to the drink "*Babycham*", of all things, during her pregnancy!

Another interesting aspect of Food Intolerance, related to time, is that the adverse reaction is not immediate as with food allergy. For example, a person can eat a food to which they are intolerant and develop symptoms over the next twenty-four to forty-eight hours. When I had a wheat intolerance, I used to develop an upset stomach within hours and then the day after I felt completely exhausted and my muscles ached, as if I had run a marathon. This makes the identification of Food Intolerance all the more difficult as often many other foods have been eaten since the problem food, so it is difficult to pin-point the exact food, or foods, which have caused the reaction.

How do you know if you have Food Intolerance?

As with Candida the range of symptoms related to Food Intolerance are many and varied. There are also remarkable overlaps, which is why, so often, people with extreme cravings and weight problems are suffering from both conditions. The complaints include:

Stomach – constipation; diarrhoea; irritable bowel syndrome; bloating, especially after eating; two sets of clothes needed for pre and post eating; indigestion; gas; heartburn.

Head – headaches; dizziness; flushed cheeks; feeling of 'sleepwalking'; feeling unreal; feeling 'spaced out'.

<u>Women</u> – Pre-Menstrual Tension (PMT); water retention; irregular periods.

<u>Blood Glucose</u> – hungry between meals; irritable or moody before meals; feeling faint/shaky when food is not eaten; irregular pulse before and after eating; headaches late morning and late afternoon; waking in the early hours and not being able to get back to sleep; abnormal cravings for sweet foods/ bread/alcohol or caffeine; eating sweets makes you more hungry; excessive appetite; instant sugar 'high' followed by fatigue; chilly feeling after eating.

<u>Mental</u> – anxiety; depression; irritability; lethargy; memory problems; loss of concentration; moodiness; nightmares; mental 'sluggishness'; "*get up and go*" has got up and gone.

<u>Other</u> – dramatic fluctuations in weight from one day to the next; easy weight gain; feeling of being unable to cope; constant fatigue; muscle aches or cramps; sighing often – 'hunger for air'; yawning easily; difficulty sleeping; excessive thirst; coated tongue; dry skin; itchiness/rashes.

Dr Brostoff uses a nice phrase, which is "*thick note syndrome.*" Where doctors see a medical file, which is thick and full of varied and seemingly unconnected complaints, they would be well advised to ask the person what they are eating.

One of the clearest signs of Food Intolerance is a huge craving for a particular food – this will be the food to which you are intolerant. The problem food produces a state of wellbeing ranging from a slight mood change to an almost manic state of euphoria. This is when the addictive aspect of Food Intolerance takes hold. Gradually more and more of the offending food is needed to produce the state of wellbeing previously provided by a normal portion of the food. At this stage, necessity is starting to replace desire. There is a *need* for the food and withdrawal symptoms will arise if the food is not eaten. For example, if you find that you get a headache mid-morning, if you don't have your usual breakfast, there may well be something that you are consuming at breakfast to which you have become intolerant.

How does Food Intolerance cause food cravings?

The real irony is that the foods to which you are intolerant are the foods that you crave. Just as the drug addict or smoker craves their fix, so you crave the substances that are causing you harm. It starts off with a particular food or drink that you consume on regular occasions. The most common offenders are dairy products and wheat, as we have them in so many different forms during the day. Any substance that we eat daily can start to cause problems and those we eat regularly, several times a day, are the chief suspects. It takes three to four days for a digested substance to pass through our bodies, so we can overload our bodies with one particular substance if we eat it daily or even more often.

Our bodies then literally become 'intolerant' to the food – i.e. they can't cope with any more of it. You would think that we would avoid a food if we had become intolerant to it, but in fact the **addiction** that goes with Food Intolerance actually means that the opposite happens. There are four stages of food addiction and we go through these stages with Food Intolerance:

- We start with an uncontrollable craving.

- We then need more and more of the offending substance in order to get the same 'high'.

- We develop physical and/or psychological dependence.

- We suffer from the adverse effects.

73

I developed a bizarre intolerance to cocoa, which resulted from over-consumption of the delicious milky coffees that I experienced when I first came across *Starbucks* ®. I found myself craving 'grande decaf lattes' to such an extent that I could easily drink four or five a day. This gave me around three pints of milk per day but ironically it was the cocoa dusting on the top that I was really craving. I found myself needing more and more each day and, if I didn't get my fix, I would get quite anxious and irritable. I realised it was the cocoa, and not the coffee or the milk, when one day there was no cocoa powder available and I realised that the froth without the powder on top did nothing to satisfy my needs. I would have an instant and significant 'high' as soon as I tasted the powder and serious withdrawal symptoms if I went without it for even a few hours.

If you want to know what you are intolerant to, simply ask yourself honestly the food(s) you would least like to give up. If you cannot imagine life without bread or cereal you should suspect wheat. If you can't face a day without eggs in any form (e.g. some pasta is egg based) then eggs could be your problem. It is so cruel, but the foods that we don't crave – those we could take or leave – are the foods that we need to keep in our diets. However, even these we need to eat in moderation and not too often as anything can become a problem if we eat it too regularly.

How can you treat Food Intolerance?

To regain control you need to identify those foods to which you are intolerant and stop eating them. You may go through intense withdrawal symptoms while you do this, but the good news is that these should last fewer than five days – just a bit more than the time it takes for a substance to pass through your body completely. You will then find that, if you eat the offending food after avoiding it for some time, you may experience extreme and sudden reactions, which is your body's way of confirming that this food is not good for you.

The key steps to treating Food Intolerance are, therefore, quite simple – find out what is causing your problems and stop eating it. Don't get depressed thinking you are about to give up some foods for life. Unlike food allergy, which remains for a life-time, Food Intolerance does come and go over time. So, you could find yourself intolerant to, say, dairy products, during a stressful period of your life when your immune system is particularly low and you may find you will be OK with dairy products again when your health is better. Many people find that they can re-introduce foods to which they have been intolerant in time, when their immunity has recovered, but only on an occasional basis. In other words, you will probably find that you can return to consuming any food or drink, in time, but you are likely to find that your symptoms and cravings reappear quite quickly as soon as you eat the substance too much or too often.

Step 1 – Identify the Foods

You can identify the foods to which you are intolerant in two main ways:

1) You can find a nutritionist or Food Intolerance practitioner to help you;

2) You can find out yourself with a bit of 'trial and error'.

1) Nutritionists and Food Intolerance practitioners use a number of ways to identify Food Intolerance. Some will just ask you to keep a food diary and then ask you questions in much the same way as the 'trial and error' method. Some will start with the most common Food Intolerance substances and eliminate these from your diet to see how you get on. Some will do skin tests or blood tests or analyse

your hair, skin and nails for signs of problems. A quite common method of diagnosis involves testing strength and pressure points by placing suspect foods on your energy lines throughout your body. An offending food placed on the energy lines will significantly impact your strength and a food that you are fine with does not. All I can suggest is for you to be open minded to whichever method your practitioner uses – they do know what they are doing.

2) With the trial and error method there are a number of things that you can try:

- The best rule of thumb is always that the foods that you crave are the ones that are most likely to be causing you problems. Anything that you eat often and in large, or increasing, quantities should be suspected. Anything that you really can't imagine **not** eating is your offending food.

- You absolutely must start a food diary, as changes can be subtle over time and it may be that you need to compare diary entries days or weeks apart to notice how far you have progressed. However, the outcome could also be quite dramatic and not at all subtle. Buy a notebook and write down everything you eat and how you feel afterwards. This alone may establish a pattern. For example, if after every entry with bread, pasta, cakes or biscuits you record that you experience bloating and stomach problems, you can start to suspect wheat as a problem.

- When you have started recording what you eat and how it makes you feel you can try to cut out the foods that you suspect and again there are a number of ways in which you can do this. You can keep your eating patterns as close to your normal eating as possible and just cut out foods that you suspect or, at the other extreme, you can start a very limited diet and re-introduce foods from there. This is when we move onto Step 2:

Step 2 – Stop eating them

When you move onto food elimination it is really important to keep that food diary going to notice any changes that do occur.

The option I recommend, to start avoiding problem foods, is to do Phase 1 of The Harcombe Diet. This eliminates all processed foods and any other foods that you suspect are causing you problems. This will give you quick results with cravings and weight loss and it is short enough a period to stick to. It will eliminate your problem foods and you can then re-introduce these, one at a time, after the five days to see how you feel. Keeping a comprehensive food diary, after every new food is re-introduced, will really help to confirm the problem foods for you.

There are two ways in which the avoidance of foods can help identify and, therefore, treat Food Intolerance. It may sound simple and obvious but when you stop eating a problem food you should feel better and when you start eating a problem food again you should feel worse. The slight complication is that initially, when you first stop eating an offending food, you may feel a lot worse and your cravings could be as bad as ever.

Remember you are craving food because you are trying to avoid the withdrawal symptoms that you get when you don't have the food to which you are intolerant. So, when you first stop eating the problem food, the withdrawal symptoms are going to come out in force. This is where the food diary will really help, as you may record feeling exhausted, lethargic and depressed and with unbearable cravings for one to five days. However, after these first few days you should feel much better. If you avoid an offending food for a few days or weeks and then go back to eating it you can suffer from quite dramatic bad symptoms. However, if you avoid an offending food for a long period of time, such as months or years, you could equally find that you have no problems with the food that previously caused you trouble.

Food Intolerance is quite a complex and sensitive area and it reflects your overall wellbeing at any one time, so it will change as you do. A food diary will really help to show what causes immediate problems (e.g. cravings, bloating) and what causes problems up to a day after (stomach upset, fatigue). You need to become highly tuned in to what you eat and how it makes you feel.

Other tips for the 'trial and error' method include:

- eat real food not processed foods. If you react badly to a cake, you won't know if sugar, wheat, eggs or dairy products are your problem as they are all in a cake. To test each substance you need to eat it on its own, e.g. to test wheat, eat shredded wheat (100% whole wheat) on its own; to test dairy products, try milk on its own; to test eggs, eat eggs on their own etc.

- eat one food at a time – one of the best ways to test foods is to avoid them for at least five days (so that there are no traces of them in your system) and then re-introduce them one by one and check for symptoms. e.g. have wheat on its own for breakfast, have only eggs for lunch and then only corn for dinner. As this is very restrictive it can be made easier by mixing one food to be tested with foods that you know don't cause you a problem. It is rare for people to be intolerant to meat, fish and vegetables so have these at each meal with just one other food that you are testing at that meal. If you suffer from symptoms, you can then be pretty sure which food has caused the problems.

- eat food a few hours apart – don't test one food within four hours of another, as the symptoms may take time to show and you could mistakenly think the second food has caused the problem. (Please note, this will help with the immediate symptoms that may develop. Your food diary will be able to help with symptoms that may develop 24-48 hours after eating a certain substance, as a pattern will emerge).

- assume the foods you most crave and would most miss are the ones causing you problems. If there are any foods that you never crave, and could happily live without, sadly these are the ones that you need to have in your diet until your Food Intolerance is brought under control.

In summary, to treat Food Intolerance you need to identify the food(s) to which you are intolerant and avoid them for as long as necessary. The complications are in the detail – how long is necessary? How do you know which foods? I hope the above section has suggested a number of ways in which you can identify your own problem foods, how you can cut them out of your diet and how you can re-introduce them to test them for confirmation.

The final stage, once your immunity and health is restored, is to eat as wide a variety of food as possible, trying not to eat any food every day and keeping a lookout for any cravings and other symptoms that could indicate that Food Intolerance has returned.

Where can we find the most common Food Intolerance substances?

The most common Food Intolerance substances can be found in so many things that we consume – from drinks to cereals. Hopefully, the following list will help you learn where to look for the thing(s) that you personally need to avoid...

Dairy Products:

Foods that always, or usually, contain dairy products include milk, cheese, yoghurt, ice cream, cream, butter, creamy pasta sauces, cakes and biscuits.

Ingredients you may see listed, which are usually dairy products, are casenin, lactalbumin, lactose and whey.

Wheat:

Foods that always, or usually, contain wheat include bread, crisp breads (unless specifically rice based), pasta, cereal, flour, pastry, biscuits and cakes.

Ingredients you may see listed, which are usually wheat based, are cereal protein, cereal binder, cereal starch, starch, edible starch and modified starch.

Corn:

Foods that always, or usually, contain corn include cornflakes, corn based cereals, corn on the cob, sweet corn and polenta.

Ingredients you may see listed, which are usually corn based, are corn meal, corn starch, corn syrup, edible starch and glucose syrup.

Eggs:

Foods that always, or usually, contain eggs include omelettes, pasta and cakes. Biscuits often contain egg based ingredients.

Ingredients you may see listed, which are usually egg based, are lecithin and ovalbumin.

<u>Soy:</u>

Foods that always, or usually, contain soy include Tofu, soy sauce, soy flour and soya bean oil. Soy products are derived from soya beans.

Ingredients you may see listed, which are usually soy based, are lecithin and vegetable protein.

<u>Peanuts:</u>

Foods that always, or usually, contain peanuts include Snickers bars, peanut butter, some cakes and biscuits. Because of genuine nut food allergies, nuts are almost always clearly identified on food packaging and in food outlets. However, these packaging alerts normally just say '*may contain nuts*' not which nuts may be present.

<u>Sugar:</u>

Foods that always, or usually, contain sugar include confectionery, biscuits, ice cream, crisp breads (many), bread (most), cereal (almost all), soups (many), salad dressings (many), pasta and cooking sauces (most), crisps (many) and prepared meals (most).

Ingredients you may see listed, which are usually sugar, are dextrose, maltose, glucose, sucrose, lactose (milk sugar), maltose, fructose and glucose syrup – anything ended in "*ose*" should be suspected as a sugar ingredient. Other ingredients to avoid are treacle, syrup, golden syrup and honey as they are processed sugars with other names.

Hopefully you will develop the view that it is far better to eat natural ingredients than packaged foods, which have up to one hundred ingredients for you to check. Why buy a pasta sauce, which almost certainly contains wheat and sugar if not dairy products as well, when you can fry some onions and garlic (great to kill off Candida), add some tomatoes (tinned with nothing added or fresh) and a few mixed herbs and you have a quick, tasty and very healthy pasta sauce.

What are food families?

Foods are grouped into 'food families'; to indicate which foods have similar characteristics and origins to each other. Food families are of interest for both Candida and Food Intolerance, as it is important to know which foods are related when you are trying to avoid foods that are harming your health. You may avoid bread, in an attempt to avoid wheat, without realising that pasta is in the wheat family too. So, if you carry on eating pasta, when you are trying to overcome your craving for bread, you will just be feeding your craving in a related way and you will continue to crave both bread and pasta.

Below is a list of food families. A main food group, such as *"meat, fish & dairy"*, is broken down into smaller groups of foods that are in the same 'food family'. The 'Cattle' food family, for example, has lamb and beef amongst other things, but rabbit is in a food family on its own.

Meat, Fish & Dairy:

CATTLE	Beef, veal, lamb, goat, milk, cheese, yoghurt
PIG	Pork, ham, bacon
DEER	Venison
RABBIT	Rabbit
PHEASANT	Chicken, pheasant, quail, partridge
GROUSE	Grouse, turkey, guinea fowl
DUCK	Duck, goose

EGGS	Are very similar in the proteins that they contain and are, therefore, in a separate category.
FISH	Are just about all in one food family. If people are sensitive to fish, this is generally food **allergy,** rather than Food Intolerance.

Some people are sensitive to 'shellfish' and not other fish, but this generally also implies food allergy rather than Food Intolerance. Shellfish include crab, lobster, crayfish, shrimp, prawn etc.

Fruit & Nuts:

ROSE (PLUM)	Plum, prune, cherry, nectarine, almond, apricot, peach
ROSE (BERRIES)	Blackberry, strawberry, raspberry, rosehip
ROSE (APPLE)	Apple, pear
CITRUS	Orange, grapefruit, lemon, lime, tangerine, clementine, kumquats
BANANA	In a family on its own (with plantain)
PAPAYA	On its own
GRAPE	Grape, raisins, sultanas
BILBERRY	Blueberry, cranberry
PINEAPPLE	On its own
GOURD	Melon, cucumber, squash, pumpkin
CASHEW	Cashew, pistachio, mango
WALNUT	Walnuts, pecans
PALM	Coconut, dates, palm oil
CURRANT	Blackcurrant, redcurrant, gooseberry

Grains:

GRASS – 1	Wheat, rye, oats, barley
GRASS – 2	Maize (corn), sugar cane
GRASS – 3	Rice
BUCKWHEAT	On its own

Herbs & Vegetables:

BEAN & PEA	All beans, peas, alfalfa, lentils, peanuts, liquorish, senna, soya beans, chickpeas, carob & mange tout.
CABBAGE	Mustard, cabbage, cauliflower, broccoli, Brussels sprouts, turnips, horseradish, radish, cress, watercress & swede.
DAISY	Lettuce, endive, chicory, artichoke, chamomile & salsify.
ONION	Asparagus, onion, garlic, leek, shallot & chives.
CARROT	Parsley, parsnip, carrot, celery, fennel, coriander, celeriac, aniseed, dill, cumin & coriander.
POTATO	Potato, tomato, aubergine/eggplant, peppers, chilli, paprika & tobacco!
SPINACH	Beetroot, sugar beet & spinach.
CUCUMBER	Melon,cucumber, squash, pumpkin and courgette/zucchini.
FUNGI	Mushrooms & yeast.
MINT	Mint, basil, oregano, rosemary, sage & thyme.

Top tips for motivation

This is one of the easiest conditions to address. Unlike Candida, which can take weeks to get under control, you can stop the cravings that follow from Food Intolerance in a maximum of five days. It takes fewer than five days for the substance causing you problems to have totally cleared itself from your body and there will then be no reason for you to crave that substance any longer. You are likely to have tough withdrawal symptoms for the first few days, but then you will feel better than you have done for ages – mentally more alert, more energetic and clear headed.

Just think – you can be free from your Food Intolerance cravings in just five days. You can be rid of that puffy, red face that greets you each morning. You can be free from stomach bloating and digestive problems that are caused by intolerance to a particular food.

One of the best motivational tips to get you going is that you could lose pounds as soon as you stop eating a food to which you are intolerant. Food Intolerance leads to dramatic water retention. When you stop eating a food that is causing you problems you are likely to lose pounds very quickly indeed and you will find that your rings, shoes and clothes fit better than ever before.

Quick Summary on Food Intolerance

- Food **allergy** is the condition of reacting badly to certain substances – like nuts or strawberries. It can be life threatening. It is not what this chapter is about.

- Food **Intolerance** is the condition of being intolerant to a particular food or foods. It is not life threatening, but it can make you feel quite unwell in a variety of ways.

- The key cause of Food Intolerance is repeated overexposure to a certain food – having too much of it and too often.

- The symptoms of Food Intolerance are many and varied and include physical, as well as psychological, complaints.

- Food Intolerance leads to food cravings because you ironically crave the foods to which you are intolerant. In fact, a sure sign of Food Intolerance is having a substance that you crave uncontrollably and try to eat as often as possible.

- When treating Food Intolerance, you need to be aware of Food Families – if you are intolerant to one food, you may well be sensitive to foods in the same food family.

- You treat Food Intolerance quite simply by not eating the foods to which you are intolerant. You probably won't have to avoid them for ever as, when your immune system is stronger, you may well be able to tolerate them again.

5

Hypoglycaemia

What is Hypoglycaemia?

Hypoglycaemia is literally a Greek translation from "*hypo*" meaning 'under', "*glykis*" meaning 'sweet' and "*emia*" meaning 'in the blood together'. The three bits all put together mean low blood sugar.

Please note, the term 'blood sugar' is often used when talking about blood glucose. However, I will only use the term blood glucose when talking about the level of glucose found in our blood, to avoid confusion with the sugar we eat (the sugar that we put in drinks or eat in confectionery bars etc). This 'table' sugar does have an effect on our blood glucose level, but we need to keep the sugar we eat separate from what happens to our blood glucose level to avoid confusion.

Fact Box: Our blood has to keep a certain level of 'glucose' at all times. If it goes above or below the safe levels of glucose, this can be really serious – even life threatening.

Hypoglycaemia describes the state your body is in if your blood glucose levels are too low. When your blood glucose levels are too low, this is potentially life threatening and your body will try to get you to eat.

Without knowing the medical detail of high, low and normal blood glucose levels you will probably be familiar with the effects. When you eat something like a confectionery bar, biscuit or cake, you may experience a surge of energy as the glucose floods into your blood stream – literally a sugar **high**.

L o w blood glucose is what you may have experienced, often late morning, late afternoon, or soon after a sugar high, when you feel irritable, hungry, have difficulty concentrating and may even have slightly shaky hands. The body's blood glucose level is crucial to our wellbeing and it is also crucial to our desire to lose weight.

Fact Box: The main thing that triggers the pancreas to produce insulin is eating sugar and processed carbohydrates. Caffeine, allergic substances, stress and alcohol can also trigger the production of insulin.

When we eat a food with any carbohydrate in it, our blood glucose levels rise and our body releases a hormone called insulin to return our blood glucose levels back into the safe zone. When we eat a fat (anything with no carbohydrate content at all), our body doesn't have to release any insulin – because fats have no impact on our blood glucose levels.

In a Diabetic, the body doesn't make insulin when a carbohydrate is eaten, because the organ that makes insulin (the pancreas) doesn't work. This is what it means to be diabetic. This is why a Diabetic has to be really careful with what and when they eat and many have to inject themselves with insulin, or take tablets, as they need medication to keep their blood glucose at the safe levels.

It is often helpful to think of Hypoglycaemia as the 'opposite' of Diabetes. Diabetes is sometimes called "*sweet urine*" and doctors test for Diabetes by asking you to give a urine sample and then seeing if there is sugar in your sample. If there is sugar in a urine sample, and a person is diagnosed as "*Diabetic*", this means that their body has not produced insulin, to return their blood glucose level to normal, after they have eaten a carbohydrate.

With Hypoglycaemia, as the 'opposite' condition, when someone eats a carbohydrate, it is almost as if the Hypoglycaemic's body works 'too well' and they produce too much insulin in response to the carbohydrate. This invariably happens when a person has eaten processed carbohydrates and the body just doesn't know how to deal with the 'sweetness' that it detects. If you drink apple juice, the body thinks you have eaten, say, twenty apples and releases insulin to 'mop up' this amount of sweetness.

The function performed by the pancreas is probably the most delicate balancing operation performed by the body and there is increasing evidence that what we eat in the 'developed world' is disturbing this mechanism. From the caveperson era to the industrial revolution, the human diet featured meat, fish, vegetables, fruits and berries and then grains, such as wheat and rice, once they became available. The current consumption of cakes, sweets, biscuits, ice cream, sugary drinks and so on is historically unprecedented and the average body just can't cope with modern food.

If you had a very sophisticated pair of scales, capable of weighing individual grains of rice, would you put a sack of potatoes on them? This is what you are doing to your body every time you eat processed carbohydrates, if your tolerance for them is anything less than perfect.

Medical opinion is divided on how common Hypoglycaemia is and how much our modern diet is to blame. Some doctors think that there are literally millions of people undiagnosed with Hypoglycaemia. Instead they are labelled neurotic, anxious, depressed, fatigued, stressed, anti-social and moody. They may also be labelled alcoholic or bulimic if they suffer from compulsive drinking and eating, as many Hypoglycaemics do. Other doctors dismiss the condition and treat people with anti-depressants and other drugs, before trying a change in diet. Every doctor, however, must surely agree with the following:

- The blood glucose balance is absolutely crucial for a healthy body and mind. In the extreme, imbalance can be fatal;

- The blood glucose level will remain more stable, and the pancreas will have to react less, on a diet of fat/protein and vegetables than on a diet of sugar and processed foods.

If we apply the theory of Hypoglycaemia to eating disorders, consider the overeater who tries to starve for a day and becomes restless, crabby, irritable, depressed and sometimes emotionally unstable. The overeater then breaks their fast with, say, a confectionery bar and becomes hyperactive, manic, bubbly, talkative and alert for probably no more than two hours before the depression and emotional instability returns.

Psychologists, dealing with eating disorders, suggest that the overeater is depressed and unstable during the fast because they are not blotting out emotional problems by eating. When they eat they feel temporary relief and then feel guilty afterwards. Undoubtedly the overeater does feel guilty after eating, but it may be low blood glucose causing the symptoms of depression and instability rather than fundamental psychological problems. This seems to have been overlooked by doctors and psychologists to date.

Recent research has shown that **fluctuations** in blood glucose are as important to Hypoglycaemia as the **actual** level of blood glucose. If the blood glucose level falls **rapidly** below normal, symptoms include sweating, weakness, hunger, rapid beating of the heart and a feeling of fear or anxiety. If the blood glucose level falls **slowly** over a period of time, a person may experience headaches, blurred vision, mental confusion, crabbiness, irritability and incoherent speech. Then, if this fall is sustained for a period of hours, the symptoms may include outburst of temper, extreme depression, sleepiness, restlessness, negativism, emotional instability, manic behaviour and general personality disorders.

Consider how this describes the overeater who starves and binges. As the starvation starts, the blood glucose level falls slowly and the person becomes confused and unable to concentrate at work. Reactions slow down, memory and mechanical ability suffer and headaches may be extremely unpleasant ('hunger headaches'). The overeater then binges and their blood glucose level rises rapidly and then falls rapidly as insulin is released by the pancreas. This rapid fall in the blood glucose level prompts hunger, weakness and a feeling of profound anxiety. This may not be simply anxiety about having binged, but general anxiety caused by Hypoglycaemia.

What causes Hypoglycaemia?

The key cause of Hypoglycaemia is the consumption of processed carbohydrates. If you eat an apple your body normally releases the right amount of insulin to 'mop' up the glucose in your blood after eating the apple and to return your blood glucose level to normal. If it doesn't do this you are diabetic or your pancreas is not working properly (probably due to the overload you have been placing on it with the food that you normally eat). As with the example we gave above, if you drink a carton of apple juice, your body thinks you have eaten, say, twenty apples and releases the amount of insulin needed to cope with lots of apples. Because you haven't eaten twenty apples there is an excess of insulin in your body and this will have the effect of lowering your blood glucose level below normal. You are now in a state of Hypoglycaemia, by definition, as your blood glucose level is low.

So, consuming processed carbohydrates can bring on the state of Hypoglycaemia temporarily and quickly. When we say that someone has Hypoglycaemia what we are really saying is that their pancreas/insulin releasing mechanism is out of balance and that they are constantly in a state of high or low blood glucose. They are rarely at a nice, even, steady level of blood glucose. They swing from one extreme to the other and suffer the energy highs and lows that go with it. This is almost certainly as a result of long term consumption of processed carbohydrates.

Some people do seem to be able to eat processed carbohydrates and 'get away with it'. Their bodies don't seem to release too much insulin, which suggests that some people may be more susceptible to Hypoglycaemia than others. However, in the majority of people, prolonged consumption of processed carbohydrates is likely to cause Hypoglycaemia. In some people it even leads to Diabetes. People who develop Diabetes later in life, invariably had Hypoglycaemia (often people did not know that they were suffering from Hypoglycaemia before they were diagnosed as diabetic). Some people's pancreases go from producing too much insulin to not producing enough, or any at all, which is the definition of Diabetes.

Diabetes and Hypoglycaemia can both be greatly helped by following a diet that contains no processed carbohydrates whatsoever. Eating processed carbohydrates can be a cause of Hypoglycaemia and maturity onset Diabetes.

How do you know if you are affected by Hypoglycaemia?

Hypoglycaemia can be diagnosed with a glucose tolerance test, which involves a series of blood tests being taken, after a glucose drink has been drunk, to measure the person's blood glucose levels. This test is rarely offered by doctors and it may be difficult to persuade your doctor to refer you for one. The perfectly acceptable alternative is to try the diet for Hypoglycaemia and keep a food diary to notice if your symptoms improve or disappear altogether.

If you follow a low carbohydrate diet for a period of time and your symptoms improve considerably you can be pretty certain that Hypoglycaemia has been a problem for you. One of the best tests, much more readily available than a glucose tolerance test, is to do Phase 1 for five days. If you have stable energy levels, a clear head and your other symptoms of Hypoglycaemia have eased then you can be sure that Hypoglycaemia was a problem for you.

The symptoms of Hypoglycaemia include the following:

<u>Head</u> – headaches; dizziness; blurred vision; feeling of 'sleepwalking'; feeling unreal; feeling 'spaced out'.

<u>Blood Glucose</u> – hungry between meals; irritable or moody before meals; feeling faint/shaky when food is not eaten; irregular pulse before and after eating; headaches late morning and late afternoon; waking in the early hours and not being able to get back to sleep; abnormal cravings for sweets or caffeine; eating sweets increases hunger; excessive appetite; instant sugar 'high' followed by fatigue; chilly feeling after eating.

<u>Mental</u> – anxiety; depression; irritability; lethargy; memory problems; loss of concentration; moodiness; nightmares; mental 'sluggishness'; *"get up and go"* has got up and gone.

<u>Other</u> – PMT (Women); dramatic fluctuations in weight from one day to the next; exhaustion; feeling of being unable to cope; constant fatigue; excessive thirst; easy weight gain.

How does Hypoglycaemia cause food cravings?

As soon as your blood glucose level falls below normal your body will cry out for food. It will crave anything, but most likely sweet foods, to get your blood glucose level back up again. When your hands are shaking, you feel a bit sweaty, a bit light headed or even faint in extreme cases, this is your body begging you to eat. You reach for a confectionery bar and immediately feel better, almost euphoric, as your blood glucose level shoots up. However, the confectionary bar is alien to your pancreas, so your body overproduces insulin, your blood glucose level falls below normal again and the cravings continue.

This is exactly why once you start bingeing you can't stop – because your blood glucose level swings from high to below normal and as soon as it is below normal you cannot resist food so you eat and it shoots back up to high again. It is a vicious circle that so many of us go through several times a day.

Not only does Hypoglycaemia cause food cravings – it directly causes you to become overweight. When you eat carbohydrates, your body decides how much of the energy taken in is needed immediately and how much should be stored for future requirements. As your blood glucose level rises, insulin is released from the pancreas and this insulin converts some of the glucose to glycogen. (Glycogen is our energy store room). If all the glycogen storage areas are full, insulin will convert the excess to fatty tissue. This is why insulin has been called the fattening hormone.

It is in fact insulin, not calories, that makes you fat. The fewer times a day you can make your body produce insulin, the better for your weight and your health. This is another reason why the last thing you want to do is to count calories. Counting calories, as you now know, means you eat more carbohydrates and only carbohydrates cause insulin to be produced.

How can you treat Hypoglycaemia?

This is pretty simple – stop eating processed carbohydrates. Do Phase 1 for five days to confirm the diagnosis and to see just how well you can feel. Then continue to eat only wholemeal carbohydrates when you move on to Phase 2.

Before insulin was discovered, the only way that Diabetics could survive was to follow a practically zero carbohydrate diet so that the body needed no insulin. Hypoglycaemia can be managed much more easily than this and you don't need to avoid all carbohydrates – just processed ones.

Top tips for motivation

This condition is the most serious of all three. Candida can make you feel really ill, but it is not life threatening. Food Intolerance, similarly, can make you feel most unwell but it is food **allergy** that is life threatening, not Food **Intolerance**. Hypoglycaemia is potentially very serious. It can lead to Diabetes, which is the fourth leading cause of death in most developed countries, third in the US. At the very least, Hypoglycaemia is your body's way of telling you that something is wrong. It is telling you that your pancreas cannot cope with what you are putting into your body and your pancreas is a vital organ for health and wellbeing.

If you care at all about your health, if the thought of possibly becoming diabetic and injecting insulin once or twice a day frightens you, then take this early warning very seriously.

This is not just about weight – your whole health and body functions are at stake here. You simply must start being kind to your body by giving it food to nourish it rather than bombarding it with junk.

Quick Summary on Hypoglycaemia

- Hypoglycaemia literally means low blood glucose.

- Hypoglycaemia is primarily caused by the over-consumption of processed carbohydrates. Some people appear to be more susceptible to it than others, but Hypoglycaemia is now believed to be very widespread.

- The symptoms of Hypoglycaemia are many and varied and include physical as well as psychological complaints.

- Hypoglycaemia leads to food cravings because when your blood glucose level falls below normal, as a result of too much insulin being released, your body will beg you to eat to raise your blood glucose level again. If you eat something else that will result in too much insulin being produced (a processed carbohydrate), your blood glucose level will fall below normal again and you will be in a vicious cycle of food craving.

- You treat Hypoglycaemia quite simply by not eating processed carbohydrates. Some people find that they need to limit all carbohydrates, until their insulin mechanism retunes, but usually people can eat wholemeal carbohydrates safely.

Part 4

The Harcombe Diet

Part 4

An Introduction

As outlined in Part 1, the five characteristics of a successful diet are:

1) It must work – and not just in the short term. It must help you reach your natural weight and stay there.

2) It must be practical – a real diet for the real world. No working out grams of protein or counting calories or carbohydrates – some simple rules that you can follow at home, at work or eating out, as part of your busy lifestyle.

3) It must be something you can follow for life – a real lifestyle change – something you can stick to easily and not something you go on and then go off leading to life-long weight fluctuations.

4) It must be healthy – and deliver the nutrients you need for healthy living.

5) It must be enjoyable – and not take away eating as a pleasure in life.

All the research behind The Harcombe Diet has shown that (1) to (5) above can **only** be achieved if you are not craving food and this, in turn, can only happen if you overcome Candida, Food Intolerance and Hypoglycaemia. So, The Harcombe Diet has three Phases:

Phase 1 (just five days long) is designed to do the following:

- To 'kick-start' your new way of eating with a programme that is short enough to stick to, but long enough to have a significant impact on Candida, Food Intolerance and Hypoglycaemia.

- To attack food cravings head on (by attacking Candida, Food Intolerance and Hypoglycaemia head on) when motivation and willpower are highest, at the start of a new diet.

- To achieve significant weight loss.

Phase 2 (for as long as you want to lose weight) is designed to do the following:

- To continue to win the war against Candida, Food Intolerance and Hypoglycaemia (and so to have continued impact on food cravings).

- To continue the great start made in Phase 1, but with a more varied diet, which is easier to stick to and more enjoyable.

- To change your eating habits forever. To get you eating real food and nourishing your body and to put you off processed foods and 'junk' as much as possible.

Phase 3 (for as long as you want to maintain your weight) is designed to do the following:

- To put you back in control of your eating by giving you long-term control over food cravings.

- To enable you to eat, without cravings, for life.

- To enable you to eat whatever you want, **almost** whenever you want, but with you managing the outcome.

6

Phase 1

Introduction

Phase 1 goes back to basics and assumes that you have any one, or all, of Candida, Food Intolerance and Hypoglycaemia. Phase 1 was developed to ensure that you only have foods and drinks that are fine for all three conditions, so that you start to attack the causes of overeating head on. It should come as no surprise that this is very similar to the diet that we would have eaten naturally, hundreds or thousands of years ago, before these conditions came about.

WHAT can you eat and drink/not eat or drink?

Meat:

As much as you want of pure, unprocessed, fresh meat – no smoked meat. This can include pork, bacon, fresh ham (i.e. with no sugars or other added ingredients), beef, veal, rabbit, chicken, turkey, pheasant, quail, goose, guinea fowl, duck, lamb, venison. Please check all ingredients, as packaged and tinned meats usually have sugars and other processed things in them.

Fish:

As much as you want of pure, unprocessed, fresh fish – no smoked fish. This can include white fish like plaice, haddock, turbot, and halibut and so on. It can include oily fish like mackerel, pilchards, tuna, and salmon and so on. It can include shellfish and seafood like prawns, lobster (provided of course that you don't have a food **allergy** to any fish or seafood).

You can eat tinned fish that has no added ingredients other than oil or salt. You can cook fish in olive oil or butter or steam, bake or grill it.

Eggs:

As many eggs as you want **if you are not intolerant to them**. They can be chicken, duck or any other eggs you can get hold of.

Tofu:

This is a Vegetarian protein alternative, which is fine in Phase 1, provided that it doesn't contain added ingredients. Take care with Tofu, because you might be intolerant to it. Soy is one of the most common Food Intolerances, in the US, and Tofu is made from the soy bean. If you have hardly ever eaten Tofu before, you should be fine and are unlikely to have developed an intolerance to it.

Salads & Vegetables:

- Salad ingredients – alfalfa, bean sprouts, beetroot, celery, chicory, cress, cucumber, endive, all types of lettuce, radish, rocket, spring onions and a couple of fruits – olives and tomatoes.

- Vegetables – artichoke, asparagus, aubergine/ eggplant, bamboo shoots, broccoli, Brussels sprouts, cabbage, carrot, cauliflower, celeriac, chillies, courgettes/zucchini, garlic, green/French beans, kale, leek, mange tout, marrow, okra, onions, parsnip, peas, peppers (any colour), pumpkin, salsify, shallots, spinach, squashes, swede, turnip, water chestnuts.

- Any herbs, spices or seasoning – basil, bay leaves, caraway, cardamom, coriander, chervil, chives, cinnamon, cloves, cumin, dill, fennel, ginger, marjoram, mint, nutmeg, oregano, paprika, parsley, pepper, rosemary, saffron, sage, salt, tarragon, thyme, turmeric.

The key vegetables that are **not** allowed are mushrooms and potatoes. Mushrooms feed Candida, so should be avoided in Phase 1. Potatoes are too high in carbohydrate for Phase 1 and they could cause problems with Candida and Hypoglycaemia as a result.

Be as adventurous as you can with salads and vegetables during Phase 1 (and Phase 2). You can make home-made coleslaw with cabbage (red and white), carrots, onions, celery and whatever else you fancy and you can use olive oil and/or beaten eggs as a dressing. You can stir-fry vegetables in olive oil and have a Chinese stir-fry with your brown rice or have a tomato/onion/garlic based sauce for your rice or meat dishes. Make Phase 1 as varied and enjoyable as you possibly can.

Brown rice:

You can have up to 50g (dry weight – before cooking) of whole-grain brown rice per day. If you are Vegetarian, or Vegan, you can have up to 150g (dry weight before cooking) of brown rice per day to make sure that you get enough to eat.

A couple of the menu options have 100g of brown rice cereal. The brand I know is called "Kallo®". I've seen it in the organic section in supermarkets and health food shops – it is 100% whole brown rice cooked into puffed pieces to make a cereal. It tastes delicious – like sugar puffs without the sickly sweet taste. Obviously don't add anything – milk or sugar – but it does taste great on its own. It has a higher glycaemic index than natural brown rice, so choose a different breakfast option if you are highly carbohydrate sensitive.

100g of cereal is equivalent to approximately 50g of brown rice, before it was turned into cereal, so it replaces the whole 50g brown rice allowance for meat/fish eaters and it leaves 100g (dry weight before cooking) of the brown rice allowance for Vegetarians.

(Please note, you don't have to eat the brown rice, but it will give you useful fibre and energy).

Natural Live Yoghurt (NLY):

Unless you are intolerant to dairy products you can have NLY in Phase 1. Remember from the Candida chapter, the great benefit you can get from NLY in the war on Candida. Try a goat's or sheep's version of live yoghurt, if you are sensitive to milk, as the health benefits of live yoghurt for Candida and the digestive tract are so significant.

Drinks:

You may drink as much bottled water (still or sparkling) or tap water as you like during Phase 1. You can drink herbal teas, decaffeinated tea and decaffeinated coffee.

You must not drink alcohol, fruit juices, soft drinks, canned drinks (even low calorie drinks), caffeinated products or milk. So, just to be clear, you can't have milk in tea or coffee during Phase 1.

Note:

Please note that we don't worry about mixing fats and carbohydrates in Phase 1. Phase 1 gets the results, without adding in this 'Rule' from Phase 2.

You must not eat anything that is not on the list above during Phase 1. No fruit, no wheat or grains (other than brown rice), no white rice, no sugar, no cakes, no biscuits, no confectionery, no cheese, no pickled or processed foods.

HOW long is Phase 1?

Phase 1 lasts for just five days.

Why five days? This very strict part of the diet needs to be short enough for you to stick to it, but long enough to have an effect. In just twenty-four to forty-eight hours you can make dramatic changes to your blood glucose stability. In three to four days, any substance to which you have been intolerant will have passed through your system and you will start to feel free from the cravings that this food has generated. Candida is the one condition that isn't 'fixed' in five days, but you can still make a big difference to Candida in five days. You will continue to fight Candida during Phase 2, but the very strict phase should be kept as short as possible so that you can stick to it.

You can continue Phase 1 beyond five days if you are suffering from all three conditions, have a lot of weight to lose and can identify with the majority of the symptoms in the chapters on Candida, Food Intolerance and Hypoglycaemia. However, as Phase 2 is merely an extension of Phase 1 (with more foods added for variety and nutrients) you may also be fine moving on to the next phase.

WHEN do you eat?

All the foods allowed in Phase 1 can be eaten whenever you want. It is best to get into the habit of eating three main meals a day, with in between meal snacks only if you are genuinely hungry. However, the most important thing with Phase 1 is to complete it, so eat whenever you want to, to make sure you are not hungry and can stick to the diet for the full five days.

HOW much do you eat?

As much as you want of everything on the 'allowed' list except brown rice, which should be limited to 50g (dry weight before cooking) per day for meat/fish eaters and 150g per day for Vegetarians.

You really can have a large plate of bacon and eggs for breakfast (just make sure the bacon has nothing added other than a preservative) and you can have as much meat, fish, salad and vegetables as you want for main meals.

If you need to snack between your three main meals then you can have cold meats, hard-boiled eggs, celery sticks, raw carrots, Natural Live Yoghurt or a tin of tuna – whatever it takes to keep hunger at bay.

You are likely to find that you actually don't fancy very much in the first few days, as you will be eating foods that you have little interest in – i.e. the foods that you don't crave.

WHY does Phase 1 work?

Phase 1 works because it is a diet just about perfect for Candida, Food Intolerance and Hypoglycaemia. You will have a significant impact on all three of these conditions in a very short period of time. Your weight loss during this short phase should also be dramatic and this will encourage you to move into Phase 2 totally committed to keeping control over your eating.

Phase 1 is designed to achieve the following:

- To 'kick-start' your new way of eating with a programme that is short enough to stick to but long enough to have a significant impact on Candida, Food Intolerance and Hypoglycaemia.

- To attack food cravings head on (by attacking Candida, Food Intolerance and Hypoglycaemia head on) when motivation and willpower are highest at the start of a new diet.

- To achieve significant weight loss.

The benefits of Phase 1 are:

-   It is strict when your willpower is highest – at the start of the diet;

-   It should be completely different to anything that you have tried before, which will jolt your body into action;

-   You will see dramatic weight loss in just five days, despite the fact that you will not be counting calories at all;

-   You will see your cravings subside each day – by day four or five they should be much more tolerable;

-   You will rid your body of all the foods, to which you are intolerant, that have been causing your ill health;

-   You will get your blood glucose level back under control straight away;

-   You will make a huge start in the fight against Candida – the yeast will have had a major attack in just a few days and will have started to die off. The ground work will have been done for getting your gut flora back in balance.

HOW will you feel?

You may feel fine. You may quite quickly feel better than you have done for years, as you stop putting into your body the foods that have been causing you problems. However, you do need to be aware that you may have some quite strong withdrawal symptoms and, if Candida is a big problem for you, you really can feel quite unwell during Phase 1. The bottom line is that the worse you feel during Phase 1, the more of the conditions of Candida, Food Intolerance and Hypoglycaemia you are likely to have had.

Remember the idea behind this diet is that you will cut out, for just five days, all foods that could contribute to Candida, Food Intolerance and Hypoglycaemia.

- If Candida has been your problem you will start to feel some quite dramatic and unpleasant symptoms as the Candida is killed off in your body. This reaction has been called 'Herxheimer's' reaction or 'Candida-die-off'.

- If you have suffered any Food Intolerance then you may notice immense withdrawal symptoms and quite unbelievable cravings for the first three to four days as your body misses the food. Once the offending substances have passed through your body, you will start to experience a physical wellbeing and mental clarity that you have possibly not felt in years.

- If Hypoglycaemia has been your problem then, within just twenty-four to forty-eight hours, your blood glucose level will stabilise and again you will experience a physical wellbeing and mental clarity that you have possibly not felt in years.

The next thing I can guarantee is that you will crave food. In this first five days, the Candida will be screaming at you to feed it. Every food to which you are intolerant will be calling out to you *'eat me'* and your hypoglycaemic body will be asking for a sugar high. The other thing I can guarantee is that your mind will start playing games with you.

On the first day of Phase 1, the cravings will come out in force and your mind will start making unhelpful suggestions. The key one it will make is *"go on – have the food you want today. You can start this diet thing tomorrow."* Sounds familiar? The trouble is – how is it going to be any easier tomorrow? The same excuse can be made tomorrow and the day after and the day after that and this is why you are still overeating and overweight when you have wanted to be slim for years. You have to start now. Don't waste another day of your life.

A key thing to remember is that Candida, Food Intolerance and Hypoglycaemia don't get better. They get worse by the day. So, if you do give in today and vow to start tomorrow, it will be even more difficult tomorrow. If you think today is tough, tackle it now before it gets any tougher.

Phase 1 will kick-start your life-long change in eating habits. It will be cleansing and cathartic, but it will also require all the willpower you have left to get to the end of the five days. You will essentially be going 'cold turkey' like a drug addict – not by giving up food, but by giving up the foods to which you have been addicted.

Pick the time you do this carefully, get friends and family to support if necessary. You may feel so unwell with the withdrawal symptoms and Candida-die-off that you may even be off work with 'sickness'. The die-off may lead to a worsening of your previous symptoms of Candida, particularly the foggy brain feeling, lack of concentration and muscle weakness. So don't start in the week when you have a key meeting or event to attend. A good option, if you can't afford to take time off, is to start Phase 1 on a Thursday and struggle through until the weekend, rest and recover over Saturday and Sunday and then by Monday you should be starting to feel quite a bit better.

The length of the die-off reaction depends on how bad your original yeast infection was, upon your current diet and on how well your body is able to detoxify. Usually any reaction begins within a few hours of starting an anti-Candida diet and it may last for a couple of weeks, in the worst cases, but each case is unique. It is really important to stick to the anti-

Candida diet, if you do get these symptoms, as this is proof that you have been suffering from an extreme Candida overgrowth. During the die-off you can help the detoxification process by drinking lots of water, eating lots of vegetables and salads (high fibre) and taking a vitamin and mineral supplement.

Many people will get through the five days feeling fine, but you should be warned of the worst extreme in case it happens to you and you think you are going down with the flu.

A final thought – you may benefit from speeding up the passage of foods to which you may be intolerant through your system at the start of Phase 1. Without being too graphic, if there is a food that always makes you go to the loo then this may be a good idea for the last day before you start the programme. This may be curry. I know someone for whom this is aubergine/eggplant. The faster we can work those offending foods through your system, the better. (You could even try colonic irrigation – people who have tried this report that they feel much more inclined to eat well afterwards).

Phase 1 for Flexis

Remember, flexis are those people who want 'dos' and 'don'ts' and meal options – not hard and fast rules. Below are some meal options for Phase 1.

(V) notes a meal suitable for Vegetarians;

(R) notes that the recipe for this meal is in Part 7 of this book.

Please remember that, other than the brown rice, quantities are unlimited – the key thing is to not get hungry, so that you can get through the five days.

Breakfasts:

- Bacon & eggs,

- Scrambled eggs (no milk) (R) (V) – cooked in butter and flavoured with salt and pepper as desired,

- Plain (V) or ham Omelette (no milk) (R) – cooked in butter and flavoured with salt and pepper as desired,

- Natural Live Yoghurt (V) (you can have a few sunflower, or other, seeds mixed in),

- Kedgeree (fish and brown rice).

Main meals (lunch/dinner):

- Asparagus in butter (V),

- Char grilled Vegetables (R) (V),

- Vegetable kebabs (R) (V),

- A selection of soups (V),

- Salade Niçoise (R),

- Salmon Niçoise (R),

- Any amount of meat & salad/vegetables,

- Any amount of fish or seafood & salad/vegetables,

- Omelette & salad (R) (V),

- Egg (V) and/or cold meat salad,

- Meat & stir-fry vegetables (R for the stir-fry),

- Tofu & vegetables in home-made tomato sauce (R for the tomato sauce) (V),

- Roast leg of lamb with rosemary & vegetables (R),

- Roast chicken with garlic or lemon (R),

- Stuffed tomatoes (R) (V),

- Stuffed peppers (R) (V),
- Brown rice with stir-fry vegetables (R for the stir-fry) (V),
- Tofu & stir-fry vegetables (R for the stir-fry) (V),
- Butternut squash curry & brown rice (R) (V),
- Paella (R) (Can be V)
- Aubergine/eggplant boats (R, V) (use the recipe in Part 7 and leave out the cheese for Phase 1).

Drinks:

You may drink as much bottled water (still or sparkling) or tap water as you like during Phase 1. You can drink herbal teas, decaffeinated tea and coffee.

Phase 1 for Planners

Phase 1 for planners has been designed to give you balance and variety throughout the five days. In this first menu plan, for meat and fish eaters, you will be having meat/fish at least once a day, eggs and Natural Live Yoghurt (NLY) once a day – more often if you have them for snacks. You also have your brown rice allowance built in. Please remember that, other than the brown rice, quantities are **UN**limited. I've tried to keep this as simple as possible – so there are no complex recipes for carnivore planners.

If you don't like eggs, or fish, or red meat, just swap in any other breakfast or main meal from the flexi list to replace this meal. You can have bacon and eggs for every one of the five breakfasts, for example. Just as you can have Chef's salad for every lunch every day, if you want. Phase 1 is only for five days, so the key thing is to find a five-day plan that works for you.

Phase 1 for Planners

DAY 1:

Breakfast	Bacon & Eggs
Lunch	Salade Niçoise (R); Natural Live Yoghurt (NLY)
Dinner	Chicken & stir-fry vegetables (R) & brown rice
Snacks	(if needed) – NLY; Crudités (sticks of carrots, celery, peppers etc); hard-boiled eggs; extra meat or fish.

DAY 2:

Breakfast	NLY OR 100g Brown rice cereal
Lunch	Plain or Ham Omelette (R – for a no milk version); Mixed salad
Dinner	Fresh salmon starter; Steak & selection of vegetables
Snacks	(if needed) – NLY; Crudités; hard-boiled eggs; extra meat or fish.

DAY 3:

Breakfast	Scrambled eggs (R – for a no milk version)
Lunch	Cold cuts of meat & brown rice salad
Dinner	Roast leg of lamb with rosemary & vegetables (R); NLY
Snacks	(if needed) – NLY; Crudités; hard-boiled eggs; extra meat or fish.

DAY 4:

Breakfast   Haddock in butter (like kipper but not smoked) OR 100g Brown rice cereal

Lunch   Chef's salad (R); NLY

Dinner   Pork chops OR salmon steaks & selection of vegetables

Snacks   (if needed) – NLY; Crudités; hard-boiled eggs; extra meat or fish.

DAY 5:

Breakfast   Plain or Ham Omelette (R – for a no milk version)

Lunch   Roast chicken with vegetables or salad; cole slaw (R); NLY

Dinner   Paella - brown rice, Mediterranean vegetables & seafood (R)

Snacks   (if needed) – NLY; Crudités; hard-boiled eggs; extra meat or fish.

You may drink as much bottled water (still or sparkling) or tap water as you like during Phase 1. You can drink herbal teas, decaffeinated tea and coffee (no milk, of course).

You may have any soup, free from wheat, sugar and dairy, with any main meal. Lots of options can be found in *The Harcombe Diet Recipe Book*.

Replace any meal that you don't like with any other breakfast or main meal from the flexi list. Have the same breakfast and main meals every day, if this works for you.

Phase 1 for Vegetarian Planners

DAY 1:

Breakfast Natural Live Yoghurt

Lunch Hard-boiled Egg salad; Natural Live Yoghurt (NLY)

Dinner Brown rice & stir-fry vegetables (R) (with Tofu – optional)

Snacks (if needed) – rest of brown rice allowance; NLY, Crudités (sticks of carrots, celery, peppers etc); hard-boiled eggs

----

DAY 2:

Breakfast Scrambled Eggs (R – for a no milk version)

Lunch Brown rice salad; Cole Slaw; NLY

Dinner Butternut squash curry & brown rice (R)

Snacks (if needed) – rest of brown rice allowance; NLY, Crudités; hard-boiled eggs

----

DAY 3:

Breakfast 100g Brown rice cereal

Lunch Omelette (R); Crudités & salad; NLY

Dinner Stuffed Peppers & Tomatoes (R); selection of vegetables

Snacks (if needed) – rest of brown rice allowance; NLY, Crudités; hard-boiled eggs

----

DAY 4:

Breakfast   Plain Omelette (R)

Lunch   Char grilled vegetables (R) with brown rice; NLY

Dinner   Brown rice, Tofu & vegetables in tomato sauce (R)

Snacks   (if needed) – rest of brown rice allowance; NLY, Crudités; hard-boiled eggs

----

DAY 5

Breakfast   Soft boiled eggs with Crudité soldiers

Lunch   Aubergine boats (R); NLY

Dinner   Vegetable kebabs (R) with brown rice

Snacks   (if needed) – rest of brown rice allowance; NLY, Crudités; hard-boiled eggs

----

You may drink as much bottled water (still or sparkling) or tap water as you like during Phase 1. You can drink herbal teas, decaffeinated tea and coffee (no milk, of course).

You may have any vegetarian soup, free from wheat, sugar and dairy, with any main meal. Lots of options can be found in *The Harcombe Diet Recipe Book*.

Replace any meal that you don't like with any other breakfast or main meal from the flexi list. Have the same breakfast and main meals every day, if this works for you.

Top tips for motivation

This is just five short days that could change your life for ever.

You will make a dramatic difference to all the conditions of Candida, Food Intolerance and Hypoglycaemia during even this brief time.

You will balance your blood glucose level and, therefore, have a huge impact on Hypoglycaemia.

You will rid your body of all the foods to which you have become intolerant.

You will make a great start in the attack on Candida to get this hideous parasite back under control in your body.

If you feel dreadful at all during the five days, this is a fantastic sign that you have had quite significant problems with the three conditions and you are making real progress.

If you feel OK, then be thankful that you have caught these conditions before they have become really bad.

No matter how you feel during the five days, you will have a clear head and mental clarity at the end of the five days that you may not have had for years.

You have to do this some time so you may as well do it now. The longer you leave it, the worse the conditions will become and the nastier the five day onslaught will be when you finally do get round to it.

Quick Summary of Phase 1

- **Do eat** meat, fish, eggs, (Tofu – if you are tolerant to soy products), Natural Live Yoghurt, any salads, any vegetables (except potatoes or mushrooms), some brown rice, herbs and spices, olive oil and butter.

- **Do drink** still or sparkling water, herbal teas, decaffeinated tea or coffee.

- **Don't eat** anything that is not on the list above. No fruit, no wheat or grains other than brown rice, no white rice, no sugar, no cakes, no biscuits, no confectionery, no cheese, no pickled or processed foods.

- **Don't drink** alcohol, fruit juices, soft drinks, low calorie soft drinks, caffeinated products or milk.

- Follow all of the above for just five days.

- Eat whenever you want – three meals a day is ideal but the key thing is not to get hungry.

- Eat as much as you want of everything on the 'allowed' list except brown rice, which is restricted.

- Do this because you are following just about the perfect diet for all three of Candida, Food Intolerance and Hypoglycaemia.

- During the five days you may feel great, you may feel fine, you may feel pretty rough. The key thing is that by the end of the five days you should be starting to feel better than you have for years.

7

Phase 2

Introduction

The key thing about Phase 2 is that it has to be workable. I have read all the diet books, just like you have, that say you must eat 2oz of home-made muesli and half a glass of skimmed milk at breakfast with chopped dried fruit pieces; a quarter cup of cottage cheese and half an apple for a mid morning snack; pan seared chicken with pasta salad and two tablespoons of home-made dressing and sautéed red snapper on black bean relish for dinner, with the recipe page references everywhere. Where is the person who can make this work for them? Everyone I know is struggling with a job, a family, studying, or all three. I don't know anyone who even has the time to shop this prescriptively, let alone do all the preparation and then eat it at the right time on the right day.

We have to be pragmatic and recognise that we all lead incredibly busy lives and we just don't have the time, or the energy, to be this black and white about our eating. What we need then are some general guidelines, which should tell us what to eat and what not to eat, but as little as possible about when and how and in what quantities.

WHAT can you eat and drink/not eat or drink

Phase 2 has just three rules. Get to know them as well as you do your best friend, as these are going to be your secret to a life-long way of eating healthily and staying at your natural weight. The three rules are:

1) Don't eat processed foods;

2) Don't eat fats and carbohydrates at the same meal;

3) Don't eat foods that cause **your** cravings.

I have seen diet books with over twenty rules, which are just far too many for any of us to take on board. None of us would ever succeed with twenty New Year's resolutions and the same applies to a change in eating habits. The three rules above are all that you need to get in control and stay in control of your eating and to reach and stay at your natural weight. Stick them on your fridge, put them in your wallet – do whatever it takes to get them ingrained in your mind.

RULE NUMBER 1

Don't eat processed foods.

From now on, you are going to eat real food. You are going to avoid any processed foods. This means:

- don't eat sugar in any form – white or brown. Anything with syrup in the title or "*ose*" at the end is usually sugar e.g. sucrose, glucose syrup, corn syrup, maltose, fructose, dextrose etc. Please note, sugar is in cakes, biscuits, confectionery, almost every cereal, most crisp breads, ready meals, many crisps, most desserts and many types of yoghurt.

- don't eat white rice, (as this is processed brown rice).

- don't eat white pasta, (as this is processed wholemeal pasta).

- don't eat white bread, as this is processed wholemeal bread (also no wholemeal bread with any processed ingredients like sugar, honey or treacle).

- don't drink fruit juice, (as fruit juice is just processed real fruit).

- don't eat dried fruit, (as dried fruit is also processed real fruit).

- don't eat chips, crisps, fries (as these are processed potatoes).

Look out for sugar, especially, in the most unexpected places. Spend an extra hour in a supermarket one day and read every label of the products you normally buy – you will be astonished at what contains sugar. I have seen sugar in cottage cheese, dextrose in packets of ham, treacle in wholemeal bread, sugar and bread in crab fish sticks and you may find many more when you look closely.

Below is a list to show you what a real food is (good) and what a processed food is (bad):

REAL FOOD – GOOD	**PROCESSED FOOD** – BAD
Grains:	
Brown rice	White rice
Wholemeal pasta	White pasta
Wholemeal flour	White flour
Wholemeal bread (without sugar, glucose syrup, treacle or other processed things)	White bread or any bread with sugar or sugar substances in it.
Fruits:	
Any whole fruits (eating the skins where edible)	Dried fruits e.g. dates
	Fruit juices
Vegetables:	
Baked potatoes with the skins on (you can make 'chips' from potatoes with their skins on, cooked with olive oil)	Normal chips, crisps, fries
	Vegetable juices, dried vegetables (vegetable crisps)
Any other vegetables	

REAL FOOD – GOOD	**PROCESSED FOOD** – BAD
Meat:	
Any pure meat with no food processing e.g. pork chops, steak, lamb joints, carvery meat etc. Any meat from the butchers or the fresh meat counter in the grocery store	Processed meats e.g. burgers, sausages Tinned meats often have ingredients added – check the label Sliced packaged meats usually have sugar/dextrose in them
Fish:	
Any fish from the fishmongers or the fresh fish counter in the grocery store Most tinned fish is OK – tuna, salmon, sardines – check the labels	Processed fish – fish fingers, fish in breadcrumbs (contains white bread and sugar)
Sugar:	
Any sugar found naturally in whole food: fruit sugar in the whole fruit; milk sugar in milk	Any sugar white or brown; maltose, dextrose, sucrose, fructose added to products; treacle; honey etc.
Drinks:	
Water, milk, herbal teas	Canned drinks, fruit juice

The simplest way to remember real food vs. processed food is to think how nature delivers it. Oranges grow on trees, cartons of orange juice don't; fish swim in the sea, fish fingers don't – you'll soon get the idea.

RULE NUMBER 2

Don't eat fat and carbohydrate at the same meal.

Eat either a fat meal or a carbohydrate meal, but don't mix the two. The exception is that salads and green vegetables have a very small carbohydrate content and can, therefore, be eaten with either fat or carbohydrate meals. So your meals should be fat meals (e.g. meat, fish, cheese, eggs) with salad and/or green vegetables **or** carbohydrate meals (e.g. brown rice, brown pasta, baked potato) with salad and/or green vegetables. (Remember the 'things with faces' tip. Fat meals have faces and carb meals don't). Coloured vegetables, like carrots, aubergine/eggplant and butternut squash, as a general rule, have a higher carbohydrate content, so they should be eaten more cautiously with fat meals.

The other two foods to be careful of are milk and nuts. Milk and nuts contain significant amounts of carbohydrate, fat and protein. They are the only foods that have all three in substantial portions. All other foods are mostly a fat or a carbohydrate. Skimmed milk is a carbohydrate and a protein with very little fat, but whole milk is also a fat. So only drink whole milk in Phase 2 with fat meals. As skimmed milk is not really a fat you can have this with wholemeal, sugar-free, cereals as a carbohydrate meal. For the same reason, don't eat nuts in Phase 2 because they are high in both carbohydrate and fat.

Here is a really useful list to show which foods can be eaten as a fat meal and which can be eaten as a carbohydrate meal and which can be eaten with either. (The *, ** and *** are explained at the end of the table):

FAT MEALS	CARB MEALS
Any unprocessed meat –bacon, beef, chicken, duck, goose, guinea fowl, ham, lamb, pheasant, pork, quail, rabbit, turkey, veal, venison.	All **Fruit**
Any unprocessed fish – cod, haddock, halibut, mackerel, plaice, pilchards, salmon, seafood *, trout, tuna, whiting etc. Includes tinned fish in only oil, salt and/or water.	**Whole-grains** – brown rice, brown pasta, brown rice pasta, 100% wholemeal bread, quinoa, millet etc.
	Wholemeal cereal – porridge oats, Brown rice cereal, Shredded Wheat, other sugar-free cereal.
Eggs – Chicken, duck etc. **	**Beans & Pulses** – lentils, broad beans, kidney beans, chick peas etc.
Dairy Products – Cheese, milk, butter, cream, yoghurt (ideally Natural Live Yoghurt)	
	Baked **Potatoes** in their skins.

EAT WITH EITHER A FAT OR CARB MEAL

Salads – alfalfa, bean sprouts, beetroot, celery, chicory, cress, cucumber, endive, all types of lettuce, radish, rocket, spring onions etc.

Vegetables – artichoke, asparagus, aubergine/eggplant, bamboo shoots, broccoli, Brussels sprouts, cabbage, carrot, cauliflower, celeriac, chillies, courgettes/zucchini, garlic, green/French beans, kale, leek, mange tout, marrow, okra, onions, parsnip, peas, peppers (any colour), pumpkin, salsify, shallots, spinach, squashes, swede, turnip, water chestnuts etc.

Tofu/Quorn – Vegetarian protein alternatives. ***

Certain **Fruits** – olives, tomatoes & berries.

Very low fat dairy products – milk, cottage cheese & yoghurt.

Herbs, Spices & Seasoning – basil, chives, coriander, cumin, dill, fennel, mint, oregano, paprika, parsley, pepper, rosemary, sage, salt, thyme. Olive oil for cooking.

* Provided of course that you don't have a food **allergy** to any fish or seafood.

** Provided that you are not intolerant to, or allergic to, eggs.

*** Provided that you are OK with vegetarian protein alternatives. Tofu is a soy product, and soy is a common Food Intolerance – especially in the US. Quorn is made from a type of fungus – so, best to avoid if you have Candida.

How to use this list:

1) You can eat anything on the 'fat' list with anything on the 'eat with either' list. You can eat anything on the 'carb' list with anything on the 'eat with either' list.

2) You should **not** eat anything on the fat and carb lists at the same meal i.e. nothing on the fat list at the same time as something on the carb list.

3) Generally, when fat is removed from a product something else needs to be put back in to replace it. The exception to this is with animal fat products where fat can be removed and nothing needs to be put back in its place. So, where there are low fat alternatives to standard products like milk and yoghurt, these low fat alternatives can be eaten with carb meals. This lets us have (very) low fat milk with wholemeal cereals and low fat cottage cheese with baked potatoes. The key is to keep fat away from carbs so carbs can be eaten with (very) low fat alternatives to dairy products.

4) You can always choose low fat dairy product alternatives to high fat ones, even when having a fat meal, and this will be beneficial for your health. However, there is nothing like being able to indulge in strawberries and cream after a grilled steak and

mixed salad, which is why this diet allows you to eat real food.

5) Some people are surprised to see any fruits on the 'eat with either' list, but olives, tomatoes and berries are low in carbohydrate relative to other fruits and so they can be eaten with either fat meals or carb meals. This makes the diet much more versatile, as it means you can have a dessert (of berries and very low fat yoghurt) after a carb meal. It also means that you can have tomato pasta sauces as well as using tomatoes in meat and fish dishes.

6) If you want to be really sophisticated about the mixing of fats and carbs then, as a rule of thumb, the more coloured vegetables are, the higher their carbohydrate content. Hence you are always safe mixing fat meals with salads and green vegetables. As you add coloured ingredients like tomatoes, beetroots, butternut squash, carrots etc, you are increasing the carbohydrate content of the meal. Hence don't mix the fattiest meat and fish you can find with the most coloured vegetables. Save green (French) beans for the roast lamb dish and use the most colourful vegetables for a chicken stir-fry.

(When people email me with queries about mixing higher carb vegetables and fat e.g. aubergine/eggplant with cheese, I go back to first principles of what this diet is all about. It is about stopping cravings and eating healthily. Fabulous as my husband's aubergine recipes are, I have never known anyone either crave them or binge on them. So, I would never worry that aubergine boats will lead to food cravings. Vegetables and cheese are natural, real foods, which provide lots of nutrients and good energy for our bodies).

I have been asked how soon after a fat meal you can have a carbohydrate meal, or vice versa. The general guideline is three to four hours, because this is how long it normally takes for food to be digested. You should achieve this naturally by having three meals a day but, if you are eating snacks, you need to leave three to four hours between eating a fat snack and a carbohydrate meal, or vice versa.

RULE NUMBER 3

Don't eat foods that cause *your* cravings.

You crave the foods that feed Candida, Food Intolerance and Hypoglycaemia and those three conditions then lead to more food cravings. You have to break out of this vicious cycle and stop eating the foods that you crave. This then helps you get rid of these conditions and you get into a positive cycle of improvement. Remember you have to stop the cravings to stop overeating. So Rule Number 3 means:

Candida – If you have a problem with Candida (you will know this from the questionnaires in Chapter 3 and from how ill you felt during Phase 1) then you will need to add the following into your Phase 2 rules:

- Limit yourself to 1-2 pieces of fruit for the first few weeks in Phase 2 – this will restrict even fruit sugar;

- Stay off wheat and bread particularly, for the first few weeks of Phase 2;

- Eat beans, pulses, brown rice and quinoa in moderation (no more than one portion a day);

- Avoid vinegar and pickled foods.

Candida is the toughest of the three conditions to have and, therefore, it has the most restricted diet to cure it. As soon as you get to the point that your Candida is feeling well under control (redo the symptoms questionnaire in Chapter 3 as a test) you can start eating more of the foods allowed in Phase 2 and eat dairy products, fruit and wholemeal grains more freely.

Food Intolerance – If there is any food to which you are intolerant, you must avoid this food in Phase 2. A great way to be sure of the food(s) to which you are intolerant is to try foods that you suspect are a problem for you **on their own** immediately after doing Phase 1.

If you eat wheat on its own for example (as plain shredded wheat cereal) after avoiding it for five days you should have a pretty rapid reaction telling you whether or not it is OK for you. If you have a return of any of the symptoms that you used to suffer from (bloating, upset stomach, headaches, for example) then you will know that this is one of your problem foods and you need to avoid it for the rest of Phase 2.

If you suspect milk, have a glass of milk on its own and see what happens. The diet for Food Intolerance is quite simple – avoid any food causing you problems. After a few weeks of avoiding the food, try it on its own and if the symptoms return you are not ready to re-introduce it. If there are no symptoms then you can eat it again, but don't have too much, or have it too often, or the intolerance will return.

Chapter 4 can also help you identify the foods to which you are intolerant, and you can then avoid these foods in Phase 2. The easiest way to identify a food to which you are intolerant is to be honest about the foods that you crave. People almost always crave the foods to which they are intolerant.

Food Intolerances do change over time, so you should find that you can re-introduce your problem foods in the future provided that you don't return to having too much of them on a regular basis.

<u>Hypoglycaemia</u> – If Hypoglycaemia is a problem for you (from the check list in Chapter 5), watch your consumption of grains and fruits as these may upset your blood glucose level. For example, in Phase 2, avoid the highest sugar fruits and don't eat more than 1-2 portions of fruit a day.

The highest sugar fruits are: bananas; melons; dates; mango; papaya; sharon fruit; pineapple – the tropical fruits.

The lowest sugar fruits are: apples; pears; peaches/nectarines; oranges; grapefruit and all berries (strawberries, raspberries, blueberries, gooseberries etc).

If there is a fruit not listed above, use the following 'rule of thumb' as to where it should go. The best fruits for you to eat are generally fruits in the supermarket all year round, like apples, pears and oranges. The fruits to eat only occasionally are tropical fruits, which are less frequently available.

If you have more than one condition you will need to follow the advice for all the conditions that affect you. This will restrict the foods that you can eat, but this is only until your immune system recovers and your body can tolerate your problem foods again. You are not giving up these foods for ever.

HOW long is Phase 2?

You should follow Phase 2 for as long as you want to lose weight. If you have a stone (14lb) or less to lose then you could easily lose 3-5lb in Phase 1 and you may only need to follow Phase 2 for a couple more weeks. If you have a lot of weight to lose then you know you can be free from hunger and food cravings throughout Phase 2 and you will lose weight whilst eating really healthy, natural foods which will be most welcome to your body.

We should note here that if you are doing well on Phase 2, and you have a special event coming up, you may like to dip into Phase 3 for a while and just maintain your weight during this occasion. The beauty of this diet is that it is so flexible you can eat in hotels and away on holiday, or at weddings, but you may want a bit more freedom for a particular occasion before reaching your natural weight. If this is the case, then read the guidelines for Phase 3 and take this ammunition along to your special occasion.

The guidelines say 1) don't cheat too much 2) don't cheat too often and 3) be alert and stay in control. If you want to eat what you like at a wedding or party, therefore, follow the Phase 2 rules right up to the minute the event starts, then eat a bit of what you fancy, but don't stuff yourself until you feel awful (i.e. don't cheat too much). Then don't look for every opportunity during the occasion to keep cheating. This means have the nice dinner, but don't eat everything at the optional, evening buffet (i.e. don't cheat too often). Finally, be alert and stay in control.

The experience will be very interesting for you to learn from – how did you feel after eating processed food? Was the way you felt worth the lapse? Treat everything as a learning experience as you get to know your body in a new, healthy way. (Please note the old 'good day/bad day' you might have starved up until the big event and then eaten everything in sight on the day and struggled to fight the bloating and tight clothes that followed. Because you no longer have 'good' days and 'bad' days, you know that a big wedding meal does not turn that day into a 'bad' day).

The other option for a special event, when you are doing Phase 2, is to go for the fat options. Eating out in restaurants, hotels or at friends' houses you will hardly ever be offered wholemeal carbohydrates. You are likely, however, to be offered meat, fish, cheese, butter and other fat options. Hence don't eat any carbohydrates that are offered (bread, potatoes and so on) and fill up on the prawn cocktail, steak, salad, cheese, cream sauces and so on and you will not have to cheat at all.

WHEN do you eat?

Eat whenever you want but you really should try to get into the habit of eating three main meals a day and only snacking in between if you are genuinely hungry.

There has been a lot of diet advice in recent years that you should 'graze' – eat little and often. I still can't believe how often I see this advice in the media. *"Keep your blood sugar level topped up throughout the day"*, is advised. Assuming that people eat carbohydrates, little and often, and not pure fat and protein, all this will achieve is that the pancreas will be overworked trying to keep your blood glucose level in the normal range. Blood glucose should be kept stable and normal to keep your body happy – any 'topping up' just has to be corrected with a dose of insulin.

Now that you know that insulin is the fattening hormone you know that the fewer times you raise your blood glucose level during the day, the better. If you graze, especially if you graze on low fat foods, which are generally high carbohydrate foods, then you are causing your body to release insulin on a more regular basis and this is what will make you fat.

HOW much do you eat?

The simple advice is – eat as much as you need. However, please be sensible. You are not tricking me if you eat until you feel sick – I will never know! You are only tricking yourself and you are not being at all nice to yourself. However much you may hate your body and, therefore, yourself, it is time to start being nice to yourself. If you don't, no-one else will. Just as you used to stuff your body, now nourish it with wonderful natural, healthy, real foods.

The key reason that this diet works so well is that you will find it almost impossible to overeat. Try eating a pound of bacon and half a dozen eggs when you can't wash it down with fruit juice or tomato sauce, or mop up the eggs with bread. Try bingeing on brown rice and stir-fry vegetables. Try overeating steak and mountains of fresh crunchy salad. Try overeating cheese when you can't have biscuits with them. Try overeating bread with no butter and when the bread is genuine wholemeal with no white flour or sugar or other processed ingredients. It will be pretty difficult – believe me.

(A small note on bread by the way – as it is such a delicious and filling food – if you are tolerant to wheat, you may like to invest in a bread maker and make your own. Recipe books come with the machines and you can throw in wholemeal flour and then add a few sunflower seeds and other tasty extras to make a really nutritious and yummy loaf. This way you can guarantee that it is free from processed ingredients).

WHY does Phase 2 work?

Phase 2 is designed to do the following:

-   To continue to win the war against Candida, Food Intolerance and Hypoglycaemia (and so to have continued impact on food cravings).

-   To continue the great start made in Phase 1, but with a more varied diet that is easier to stick to and more enjoyable.

-   To change your eating habits forever. To get you eating real food and nourishing your body and to put you off processed food and 'junk' as much as possible.

The rationale behind Phase 2 is really simple and powerful:

Rule 1 – Don't eat processed foods

This is because when you eat processed foods your body releases the amount of insulin as if you have eaten the whole food (when you drink apple juice, your body thinks you have eaten lots of apples and pumps out enough insulin to mop up lots of apples). We must stop this happening for two key reasons:

1) As insulin is the fattening hormone we want our bodies to release the right amount of insulin to mop up the food we have actually eaten, not too much, so that the extra is stored as fat. If we eat the whole apple, or whole grains, i.e. the whole food every time, our bodies should release the right amount of insulin.

2) If we end up with too much insulin, after eating something, our blood glucose level will be low, which will make us crave food to get our blood glucose level back to normal. So, we will have cravings for food – especially processed foods – which is what has made us overeat and overweight in the first place.

Processed foods are 'empty calories'. They give us calories, which provide energy/fuel, but they don't give us as many nutrients as we could get from eating the same number of calories from real food. If we don't get the nutrients we need, we will crave foods to make sure we eat the foods we need for certain nutrients. If we eat a varied diet of real food – meat, fish, eggs, dairy products, vegetables, salad, fruit, nuts, and seeds – we will be more likely to get the nutrients we need and our body won't need to crave things. If we eat microwave meals, cakes and biscuits and so on, we are going to crave nutrients.

Rule 2 – Don't eat fats and carbohydrates at the same meal.

This is for two reasons:

1) The easiest substance for the body to get energy from is carbohydrate. So, if your body spots that you've eaten a carbohydrate it says *"Thank you very much – I'll use that for my immediate energy needs and I'll store any fat with it for later on"*. The double whammy is that the body needs insulin to store fat, and it is only carbohydrates that cause insulin to be made. So your body can only store that fat, for later on, when you have eaten a carbohydrate.

   If you eat carbohydrate, and no fat, the body uses the carbs for energy and there is no fat to store. If you eat fat, and no carbohydrate, your body has to use the fat for energy and it has to work a bit harder to do this – which is good news for you, because it naturally uses up more energy. As we don't want fat to be stored, we must not eat the two food groups at the same time.

2) The second and less important reason is that the stomach produces acid based juices to digest protein/fat and the juices necessary to digest carbohydrate are alkaline. If you eat carbohydrate with protein/fat you are mixing acid juices with alkaline juices and they cancel each other out. Then neither the carbohydrate nor the protein/fat gets digested.

Rule 3 – Don't eat foods that cause *your* cravings.

You crave the foods that feed any of the three conditions, from which you may be suffering, because Candida, Food Intolerance and Hypoglycaemia all lead to unbelievable food cravings. To lose weight you have to stop the cravings. To stop the cravings you have to get these three conditions back under control.

HOW will you feel?

You should feel fantastic! You need not be hungry. You will be free from cravings. You will be eating real, healthy foods, which will be nourishing your body and giving you energy like you've not had for years. You can eat both carbohydrate and fat (just not at the same time) so you should not feel deprived. You will be able to eat out and dine in, snack and lose weight, at the same time as keeping your busy lifestyle.

Not only are you eating healthy foods, but also you are avoiding processed foods, which are unhealthy foods. So you are eating the goodies and avoiding the baddies. Most importantly you are avoiding sugar, which contains no nutrients whatsoever, and other processed foods, which have had most of their goodness removed in the processing.

In Phase 3 you will be able to choose whether or not you want to eat processed foods again. It will be interesting to see what choice you make.

Phase 2 for Flexis

Below are a number of different possible breakfasts and main meals for Phase 2 – either fat options or carbohydrate options. There is a code after each meal to indicate what the meal is suitable for:

C = suitable for Candida

H = suitable for Hypoglycaemia

P1 = suitable for Phase 1 as well as Phase 2

R = the recipe for this is in Part 7

THDRB = the recipe for this is in The Harcombe Diet Recipe Book

V = suitable for Vegetarians

It is difficult to indicate which meals are OK for sufferers of Food Intolerance, as some people may be intolerant to wheat, others to milk, others to corn and so on. If you know that there is a food to which you are intolerant then obviously don't choose the meal options that contain that food.

It is also a bit difficult to indicate which meals are OK for Hypoglycaemia as some people may be able to tolerate more fruit or grains than others. Again, please adjust the meal list according to your own needs.

Please note that you can choose whether to have a fat meal or a carb meal whenever you like – you may like every meal to be a fat meal or every meal to be a carb meal – or any combination in between. I recommend at least one fat meal and one carb meal a day for variety.

Breakfasts – fat meals

- Bacon & Eggs (C, H, P1)

- Kippers/smoked haddock (H)

- Scrambled eggs (C, H, P1, R, V)

- Plain omelette (C, H, P1, R, V)

- Ham omelette (C, H, P1, R)

- Natural Live Yoghurt (C, H, P1, V)

- Please note cooking options for fat breakfasts include grilling, poaching, steaming, baking or frying in butter or vegetable oil.

Breakfasts – carb meals

- Fruit platters (C, H, R, V)

- Fruit and very low fat natural yoghurt (C, H, V)

  (Please note, limit fruit to 1-2 portions a day, in Phase 2, if you have C and/or H)

- Shredded Wheat & milk (H, V) (with a sliced banana for sweetness – optional)

- Brown rice cereal (best on its own – as it stays crunchy) (C, H, V) (use as P1 rice allowance)

- Sugar-free porridge with water, or milk (skimmed) (C, H, V)

- Sugar-free muesli with water, or milk (skimmed) (H, V)

- Wholemeal bread & sugar-free preserves (H, V)

Main Meals – Starters – fat meals

- Prawn cocktail (C, H) (Can be OK for P1 with an egg and olive oil only mayonnaise)

- Tomatoes & Mozzarella (C, H, V)

- Asparagus in butter (C, H, P1, V)

- Salmon & cream cheese (C, H) (Avoid *smoked* salmon if you have Candida)

Main Meals – Starters – carb meals

- Char grilled vegetables with olive oil or balsamic (No balsamic vinegar for P1) (C, H, P1, R, V)

- Vegetable kebabs (C, H, P1, R,V)

- Melon selection (V) – too high in sugar for C & H

- Fruit salad (C, H, V) (Get used to having fruit before the main course & limit fruit to 1-2 portions a day, if you have C and/or H)

- A selection of soups (C, H, P1, THDRB, V)

Main Meals – Main Courses – fat meals

- Salade Niçoise (C, H, P1, R)

- Salmon Niçoise (C, H, P1, R)

- Any meat & salad/vegetables (C, H, P1)

- Any fish & salad/vegetables (C, H, P1)
- Omelette & salad (C, H, P1, V, R)
- Ham, egg, cold meat salad (C, H, P1)
- Chef's salad (C, H, R)
- Four cheese salad (C, H, R, V)
- Cheesy leeks (C, H, R, V)
- Cauliflower cheese (C, H, R, V)
- Meat & stir-fry vegetables (C, H, P1, R)
- Quorn & vegetables in tomato sauce (H, V)
- Aubergine boats (C, H, R, V) (Leave the cheese out for a P1 dish)
- Roast leg of lamb with rosemary & vegetables (C, H, P1, R)
- Roast chicken with garlic or lemon (C, H, P1, R)
- Egg & Asparagus bake (C, H, R, V)

Main Meals – Main Courses – carb meals
- Brown rice & stir-fry vegetables (C, H, P1, R, V)
- Quinoa with stir-fry vegetables (C, H, R, V)
- Wholemeal pasta & tomato sauce (H, R, V)
- Wholemeal spaghetti & tomato sauce (H, R, V)
- Vegetarian chilli and brown rice (C, H, R, V)
- Couscous & Char grilled vegetables (C, H, R, V)
- Butternut squash curry & brown rice (C, H, P1, R, V)
- Baked potato & salad and/or very low fat cottage cheese (C, H, V)
- Roasted vegetables with pine nuts & Parmesan cheese (C, H, R, V)

- Stuffed tomatoes (C, H, P1, R, V)

- Stuffed peppers (C, H, P1, R, V)

There are many more recipes for carb main courses in *The Harcombe Diet Recipe Book* e.g. Lentil Moussaka, couscous & chickpeas in coriander sauce and Basil & Pine nut quinoa.

Main Meals – Desserts – fat meals

- Strawberries & Cream (C, H, V)

- Sugar-free ice cream (C, H, THDRB, V)

- Natural Live Yoghurt (C, H, P1, V)

- Greek Yoghurt (C, H, V) (Can be full fat with a fat meal)

- Cheese selection (C, H, V)

Main Meals – Desserts – carb meals

- Any berries with very low fat yoghurt (e.g. strawberries, raspberries, blackberries etc) (C, H, V)

- Berry compote (C, H, THDRB, V)

- Fruit puree (C, H, THDRB, V)

- Fruit salad (C, H, V)

(Please remember to limit all fruit to 1-2 pieces a day if you have C and/or H)

Easy Lunches for Work – fat meals

- Tinned tuna/salmon with salad in a lunch box (C, H, P1)

- Cuts of cold meat (chicken, turkey, beef, ham – any combination) with salad (C, H, P1)

- Any fat leftovers from dinner the night before.

Easy Lunches for Work – carb meals

- Brown bread salad sandwich (H, V)
- Brown rice salad – cold brown rice with chopped salad ingredients (C, H, P1, V)
- Any carb leftovers from dinner the night before.
- Baked potato * & salad and/or very low fat cottage cheese (C, H, V)
- Fruit salad * (C, H, V)

* Remember to take care with high carbohydrates, such as potatoes or fruit, with Hypoglycaemia.

Snacks – fat options

- Cheese (C, H, V)
- Hard-boiled eggs (C, H, P1, V)
- Natural Live Yoghurt (C, H, P1, V)
- Cold cuts of meat (C, H, P1)

Snacks – carb options

- Sugar-free cereal bars – ideally go for a wheat-free one also. Health food shops have a reasonable selection (H, V)
- Sugar-free oat biscuits (C, H, V)
- Fruit (C, H, V)
- Rice cakes (V) – not ideal for C and H, as they have a high glycaemic index

Snacks – either

- Crudités (sticks of carrots, celery, peppers etc) (C, H, P1, V)

Phase 2 for Planners

Phase 2 for planners has been designed to give you balance and variety in a weekly plan, which you can repeat week after week for as long as you need to lose weight.

This 7-day menu plan is the purest version of The Harcombe Diet. It assumes that you have Candida, wheat Food Intolerance and Hypoglycaemia and excludes the foods that you should avoid for each of these.

This 'pure' version of the diet also shows how to have snacks in between fat and carb meals, so that you don't mix fats and carbs. It is ideal to **try to avoid snacks**, and get used to eating three large meals a day, but the following has allowed for snacks morning and afternoon, if you feel you can't do without snacks.

The shaded lines below are fat meals and the non-shaded lines are carb meals. You can swap in any fat or carb meal, from the flexi list, whenever you like, to add variety and to avoid something that you may not like. You can add any carb starters or desserts from the flexi list to carb meals and add any fat starters or desserts from the flexi list to fat meals. Please remember that, other than the pieces of fruit specified, quantities are unlimited.

DAY 1:

Breakfast	Bacon & Eggs
AM snack	Natural Live Yoghurt (NLY)
Lunch	Salade Niçoise (R)
PM Snack	1-2 pieces of (lower sugar) fruits
Dinner	Butternut squash curry & brown rice (R)

DAY 2:

Breakfast   Porridge with water (or skimmed milk, if no dairy intolerance)

AM snack   1-2 pieces of (lower sugar) fruits

Lunch   Roasted Vegetable Salad (R)

PM Snack   NLY

Dinner   Roast chicken (R) with vegetables & salad

DAY 3:

Breakfast   NLY

AM snack   Hard-boiled egg and/or NLY

Lunch   Chef's salad (R)

PM Snack   1-2 pieces of (lower sugar) fruits

Dinner   Brown rice & stir-fry vegetables (& Tofu – optional)

DAY 4:

Breakfast   Brown rice cereal

AM snack   1-2 pieces of (lower sugar) fruits

Lunch   Baked potato & low fat cottage cheese or low fat natural Live Yoghurt or ratatouille (R)

PM Snack   NLY

Dinner   Pork or Lamb chops or salmon steaks with vegetables & salad

----

DAY 5

Breakfast	Scrambled eggs (R) (with milk, if no dairy intolerance)
AM snack	NLY
Lunch	Baked, poached, grilled, fried or steamed fish & vegetables
PM Snack	1-2 pieces of (lower sugar) fruits
Dinner	Rice pasta in 15 minute tomato sauce (R)

DAY 6

Breakfast	Porridge with water (or skimmed milk, if no dairy intolerance)
AM snack	1-2 pieces of (lower sugar) fruits
Lunch	Char grilled vegetables (R) & brown rice
PM Snack	NLY
Dinner	Steak & Mixed Grill or a large fish like trout or mackerel

----

DAY 7

Breakfast	Plain or ham omelette (with cheese, if no dairy intolerance)
AM snack	NLY
Lunch	Roast lamb, pork, beef or chicken. Selection of vegetables
PM Snack	1-2 pieces of (lower sugar) fruits
Dinner	Vegetarian chilli & brown rice (R)

Phase 2 for Vegetarian Planners

Phase 2 for Vegetarian planners, like the Phase 2 for non-Vegetarian planners, assumes that you have Candida, wheat Food Intolerance and Hypoglycaemia and excludes the foods that you should avoid for each of these. Please remember that, other than the pieces of fruit specified, quantities are unlimited.

This 'pure' version of the diet also builds in snacks and it plans fat and carb meals in the right order, so that not mixing fats and carbs is sorted for you. It is ideal to **try to avoid snacks**, and get used to eating three large meals a day, but the following has allowed for snacks morning and afternoon.

The shaded lines below are fat meals and the non-shaded lines are carb meals. You can swap in any fat or carb meal, from the flexi list, whenever you like, to add variety and to avoid something that you may not like. You can also add any carb starters or desserts from the flexi list to carb meals and add any fat starters or desserts from the flexi list to fat meals.

DAY 1:

Breakfast	Porridge with water (or skimmed milk, if no dairy intolerance)
AM snack	1-2 pieces of (lower sugar) fruits
Lunch	Stuffed Peppers/Tomatoes (R)
PM Snack	Natural Live Yoghurt
Dinner	Egg & Asparagus bake (R)

DAY 2:

Breakfast	Scrambled eggs (R)
AM snack	Natural Live Yoghurt
Lunch	Four cheese salad (R)
PM Snack	1-2 pieces of (lower sugar) fruits
Dinner	Stir-fry vegetables & brown rice

DAY 3:

Breakfast	Puffed rice cereal
AM snack	1-2 pieces of (lower sugar) fruits
Lunch	Baked potato & low fat cottage cheese or low fat natural Live Yoghurt or ratatouille (R)
PM Snack	Natural Live Yoghurt
Dinner	Cheesy leeks (R)

DAY 4:

Breakfast	Natural Live Yoghurt
AM snack	Hard-boiled egg and/or crudités
Lunch	Omelette (R) & Salad
PM Snack	1-2 pieces of (lower sugar) fruits
Dinner	Butternut squash curry & brown rice (R)

144

DAY 5

Breakfast   Porridge with water (or skimmed milk, if no dairy intolerance)

AM snack   1-2 pieces of (lower sugar) fruits

Lunch   Char grilled vegetables (R) & brown rice

PM Snack   Natural Live Yoghurt

Dinner   Aubergine boats (R)

DAY 6

Breakfast   Plain omelette (with cheese, if no dairy intolerance)

AM snack   Natural Live Yoghurt

Lunch   Cauliflower cheese (R)

PM Snack   1-2 pieces of (lower sugar) fruits

Dinner   Vegetarian chilli & brown rice (R)

DAY 7

Breakfast   Fruit platter with low fat Natural Live Yoghurt and/or cottage cheese

AM snack   1-2 oat biscuits (oats, oil & salt – no other ingredients)

Lunch   Rice pasta in 15 minute tomato sauce (R)

PM Snack   Hard-boiled egg and/or crudités

Dinner   Four cheese salad (R)

Coffee and Wine

Just a final word on drinks in this 'what do you eat' section...

We have said that this diet must be workable, so there are two areas where you can 'cheat' in Phase 2 to help it work for you:

1) There are some people who just cannot face the thought of starting the day without an espresso or regular coffee or a cup of tea. There are a number of points to make here:

   - Take care that it really is the coffee/tea that you are so keen to have and not a craving for milk, which could be a sign of milk Food Intolerance.

   - Try to switch to decaffeinated alternatives if at all possible.

   - If you are not craving milk, you loathe decaf. and you really want that first espresso of the day, then have it. The key thing is that you stick to this diet so, if a coffee or a cup of tea in the morning would make the difference between you sticking to this diet or giving up, then have one.

   - However, make sure you don't go over one, maximum two, cup(s) a day. Ideally have them before early afternoon; otherwise they will disturb your sleep patterns later that night.

   - Have your early morning coffee with a carbohydrate breakfast, rather than a fat breakfast, as the caffeine will raise your blood glucose level and you don't want that insulin in your body looking for a fat breakfast to store.

   - Be aware that caffeine will give you a short term high followed by an energy low so have a strategy for getting your blood glucose level back to normal. One case study I worked with had his espresso as soon as he woke up and then had his sugar-free muesli with milk after showering, so that the healthy breakfast naturally raised his blood glucose level back to normal after the caffeine high.

2) The other thing that some people just can't do without is a glass of wine with dinner. There are similar points to make here too:

- Take care that you are not craving the specific ingredients in wine and feeding Candida and/or a specific Food Intolerance. If Candida is a problem for you then you must avoid wine until this condition is back under control.

- Try to drink dry and organic wines as much as possible to limit the sweetness and additives that you consume.

- If this will make the difference with you sticking to the diet then have an occasional glass of wine, ideally red, with your main meal of the day.

It is obviously better in Phase 2 not to drink caffeine or wine, but the key thing is to stick to the diet.

Top tips for healthy eating:

There are only three rules in Phase 2 and these are by far and away the most important things to take out of this book. Following just these three rules can change your eating and weight for ever. There are, however, some other things that you can do to optimise your health and the way in which you eat. If you do any of these already, well done – keep it up. If not, you may like to try to add another one each month but only when Rules 1-3 are completely second nature to you.

The other good things that you can do are:

1) Don't go hungry;

2) Do eat fruit *before* other foods;

3) Do drink plenty of water *between* meals (1.5 litres per day);

4) Don't drink *with* meals (with the exception of the odd glass of wine – especially red).

The tips above are about healthy eating, not weight loss. However, they all have implications for weight loss, so they are worth knowing about.

1) If you are hungry you are more likely to crave food as your body will cry out for anything to stop the hunger. So don't go hungry or you will invite hunger pangs and cravings to return.

2) If you eat fruit after other foods, especially meat and fish that take much longer to digest, the fruit gets stuck behind the other foods in your digestive tract and this is one of the causes of stomach bloating. This can have an impact on losing weight a) because the fruit is not able to be properly digested by the body and b) because the bloating will make you feel fat and then you may be tempted to eat more – because you already feel fat, so you may as well.

3) If you drink lots of water between meals, your body can rid itself of waste products more easily and all your organs, such as the liver and kidneys, can do their jobs much better. Water also stops hunger pangs because often people are thirsty, not hungry, when they want food. (There is so much water in food that food naturally quenches our thirst – fruits especially). Drinking lots of water also makes you feel energetic and healthy and it is great for your skin and hair. When you feel good you want to make the effort to stick to your diet and look good.

4) Drinking at mealtimes floods the body's natural digestive juices and hampers the body's ability to digest the food. The better we digest food, the better it passes through our body, and so it is important not to do anything to upset the digestive process.

Quick Summary of Phase 2

1) Don't eat processed foods;

2) Don't eat fats and carbohydrates at the same meal;

3) Don't eat foods that cause *your* cravings.

- Follow all of the above for as long as you need to lose weight.

- Eat whenever you want – three meals a day is best but the key thing is not to get hungry.

- Eat as much as you want of everything on the 'allowed' list. Follow the restrictions for Candida and Hypoglycaemia advice.

- Do this because you are following just about the perfect diet for all three of Candida, Food Intolerance and Hypoglycaemia.

- During Phase 2 you will feel great, energised, nourished and free from cravings or hunger.

Top Tips for Phase 2 - NEW

Since my first book was published, I have qualified as a nutritionist, having completed a Diploma in Diet and Nutrition and a Diploma in Clinical Weight Management. Despite both courses being very interesting, I see them both, quite literally, as 'academic'. Neither can compare with the value of the personal experience gained from having had anorexia, bulimia and food addiction and from having tried every diet under the sun. I love working with the many wonderful clients that I meet and there is nothing in a nutrition course that can enable you to empathise with someone who is addicted to food, and desperate to lose weight, unless you've been in the same situation.

In this new section, I would like to share with you some of the key points that I share with clients when we work together:

1) The incredible weight loss, which many people achieve in Phase 1, is not sustainable. Much as I would love for you to lose several pounds every week, week in week out, it is extremely unlikely to happen. Candida and Food Intolerance cause significant water retention and, if you lose over half a stone in five days (as regularly happens), much of this will be water and this can only be lost once. As long as you keep these two particular conditions under control, there is no reason for this water to return, and this weight loss really does count – you can drop a clothes size, or even two, in a matter of days and look and feel so much better.

2) On the subject of water vs. fat loss, weight is weight. The human body is approximately 50% water, so you are always going to lose water as you lose weight. So long as you don't lose water in an unnatural way, with diuretics, if you are normally hydrated and you weigh less than last week, you have lost weight and you will feel and look slimmer.

3) There is no formula on earth when it comes to weight loss. The "*to lose 1lb of fat...*" formula in Chapter 2 absolutely does not work (ask the next person who says this to you where it comes from and what the evidence for it is – they won't be able to tell you). If you had found something that gave you sustained 2lb a week weight loss, you would have lost 104lbs in the past year (and the year before and the year before that) and you wouldn't be reading this book. I'm really sorry if I am the one breaking this to you, but there is no formula.

Hence, sadly, I genuinely cannot predict what your weight loss will be on The Harcombe Diet. I can share with you numerous testimonials from people who have lost a great deal of weight and kept it off. Many come to say that the weight loss is almost a bonus – what they love even more is the freedom from food addiction and cravings and the incredible energy and wellbeing that they have.

I can share that people comment time and time again that a pound lost on this diet is gone for good – because you have not slowed your metabolism, there is no tendency for you to put on weight the minute you start eating 'normally', as happens on other diets. Your whole concept of normal eating will become a lifelong commitment to nourishing your body with real food and cheating when you want to and getting away with it.

Check out Facebook, Amazon and YouTube for comments about the diet. You will find lots of inspiring stories of people who have lost stones and are wearing their target size jeans for the first time in years. Posting such as "*Bought the book, it's a super read, I have lost 2 stone 2lbs in 5 weeks*" (YouTube) make my day! Follow the rules and you will lose weight and you will keep it off. However, no one on earth can tell you how quickly you will reach your natural weight.

4) Phase 1 vs. Phase 2 is up to you. Phase 1 is the fastest weight loss plan I have come across, but Phase 2 delivers better on the practical and enjoyable characteristics of a diet. There is a trade off between faster weight loss with a more restricted plan and steadier weight loss and a more varied plan – the choice is yours and you can flex between the two from week to week, to suit your lifestyle.

5) If you did well on Phase 1 and then don't lose any weight for more than a couple of weeks in Phase 2, this can pretty much only be due to something you have re-introduced in Phase 2. You need to be quite analytical and look at everything you have added back in and see if you have added in anything that could have started to 'feed' one of the conditions. Wheat would be my first suspect. I have yet to meet someone who does not feel better and lose weight faster staying off wheat until at least close to their goal weight. Things that 'feed' Candida and Hypoglycaemia are the next suspects – fruit, whole grains – any substantial increase in carbohydrates into your diet can have an impact if you are very carb sensitive. Re-read Chapter 7 on Phase 2 and follow the advice for the three conditions really carefully to make Phase 2 work for you.

6) Plateaus – because there is no formula that can predict weight loss, there is no way of knowing how much will be lost each week. Some people do find that they plateau – even for a few weeks (this is rare), but then they suddenly start losing steadily again and a month later almost another stone has gone. Plateaus are so frustrating and my heart really does go out to people who are sticking so well to the diet and who don't get the reward that week – but the reward does come. We just can't predict when –

boy do I wish I could. I know I can take away cravings and I know that Phase 1 works for everyone who has tried it. I just can't guarantee you will lose weight every single week, week in week out.

Consider this, though: the majority of my success stories have been doing calorie controlled diets for at least 10 years and they had reached the point where they had stopped losing a single pound, despite trying to survive on 1000-1200 calories a day. They try Phase 1, lose 5-10lbs in a week and never look back. You will get there and you will be eating really healthily in the meantime and will no longer be hungry and exhausted.

7) I have developed a theory, working with clients, that weight loss is as much about overcoming fat storage as it is about encouraging fat burning. I really believe that the bodies of long term calorie counters are trained to store fat and we need to re-train the body to stop storing fat. The best way I have found for doing this is to have clients eat three substantial and nourishing meals a day and to eat these as regularly as possible. The body then knows when the next fuel is coming and quickly learns that it doesn't need to store fat any more. I am really pleasantly surprised how quickly the human body responds positively to healthy eating and how rapidly it starts to work with you.

To accompany this principle, I cannot recommend strongly enough (I do repeat this so often in the book) – limit snacking and avoid snacks altogether if at all possible. If you really are hungry between meals try to eat more at meals, so you are not hungry and/or stick to carb free snacks if possible. Whenever you eat a carbohydrate, the body goes into a glucose/insulin/fat storing environment and you want it to be in a fat burning environment, to use up your love handles. The less often you eat carbs, during the day, the better. Carbs and insulin really are the secret to weight loss.

8

Phase 3

Introduction

This chapter is the nicest gift that I can give anyone who has struggled with their weight, or been out of control with food, at any time in their life. This really is the secret of how to have your cake and eat it. If I had a dollar for every time someone has asked me how I can eat so much, or eat chocolate and ice cream, and stay so slim, I could have retired at thirty!

Please note that you should only move onto Phase 3 when you are at your 'natural' weight. The first thing to point out here is that your 'natural' weight may not end up being what you currently expect. There is much evidence that we have a natural weight, which our bodies tend towards. If we put on weight temporarily (e.g. on holiday or during festive seasons) then we will return to our natural weight when we return to normal healthy eating patterns. Similarly if we lose weight during an illness or personal upset we will return to our natural weight when we return to normal healthy eating patterns. I am 5ft 2" and my natural weight seems to be 8st (112lb). I have been below this in recent years, during times of illness or extreme personal stress, and I have gone over this when I have had phases of 'cheating' too much, too often. However, I seem to be able to stay at 8st easily.

You may find that your natural weight is not exactly where you would like it to be. Many people have an 'unnatural' goal for their weight – largely driven by painfully thin models, magazines, peer pressure and unhealthy body images. You may also find that as you exercise and lose weight simultaneously you end up with a toned, athletic shape, rather than a bony, skinny shape, which is much healthier and far more attractive.

So please be open minded about your natural weight and for this to be slightly above (or below) your current thinking on your 'ideal' weight. Please note that you may be reading this book when you are actually at your natural weight. You may just want help staying there and you may want a way out of the bingeing and starving, or calorie counting, which is probably keeping you at this weight. If this applies to you then you may like to try Phase 2 for a while, until you feel free of cravings and in control of your eating, and then you can move to Phase 3 quite quickly.

Your natural weight, remember, will be the weight that you can maintain easily – going above it takes some overeating and going below it happens when you are ill or under stress. We all have a natural weight and you will be delighted when you find yours and realise how much you can eat and still stay at this weight.

WHAT can you eat and drink/not eat or drink

You really can eat what you want **almost** when you want. This will be called 'cheating'. The key thing is to make sure that the cravings don't return and here is how you achieve this:

1) Don't 'cheat' too much;

2) Don't 'cheat' too often;

3) Be alert and stay in control.

When you end the weight loss plan you can eat anything that you want. That probably bears restating – when you no longer want to/need to lose weight you can eat anything that you want. Chocolate, ice cream, cakes, biscuits, pasta – whatever. However, what you will realise is that, whereas before you only avoided certain foods in an attempt to lose weight, you may now choose to avoid certain foods in a desire to feel well. You will get to the stage when you are at a weight you are happy with and you will be able to control your eating as your cravings will have disappeared and you will, therefore, have the choice about what you want to eat. You will be experiencing the following:

- you will no longer crave food;

- you will feel healthy and free from the many physical and emotional symptoms which were described in Part 3;

- you will be eating to live rather than living to eat;

- you will have more energy and zest for life than probably ever before;

- you will be enjoying a wide variety of healthy and nourishing foods.

The ideal way of eating for Phase 3 is to keep rule number one from Phase 2 – don't eat processed foods – and that alone. Your health will not suffer at all if you never eat another processed food again in your life. Hopefully having tasted the nutty flavour and filling texture of brown rice you will never want to return to white rice. Hopefully sugar-free multi-grain, wholemeal bread will be your natural choice over white bread any day. There is less difference between wholemeal and white pasta but hopefully the brown variety too will remain your natural choice.

You can stick with Phase 2 for life and you will live very healthily for doing so. However, if we return to the key attributes of a successful diet earlier on in the book, there may well be reasons for eating processed foods, on occasions, when your eating and weight are under control. For some people the thought of never eating confectionery or ice cream again is just too much to think about. You truly will get to the point where you can live without ice cream, but it is understandable to think that not everyone will want to do this.

Phase 3 is all about guidelines and the bottom line is to **be alert and stay in control**. You will be armed with a huge amount of knowledge as you set off on a new phase of freedom. You won't eat cartons of Haagen-Dazs ® and M&Ms ® and not understand why. You will be alert for the three conditions that lead to food cravings and you will be able to nip them in the bud the minute that they reappear.

Candida is probably the toughest to keep under control because of the rate at which yeast multiplies. You may start eating processed foods again and get away with it for days, weeks or even months and then, one day, your cravings will be back as strong as ever and the yeast will have been fed back out of control. One of the best ways to avoid this is to keep your immune system strong. Take a vitamin and mineral supplement every day, take extra vitamin C at the first sign of a cold (a sure sign of a lowered immune system), keep your life balanced and full of things that you enjoy and you will keep the best defence possible against Candida. Avoid antibiotics unless your life is threatened. Avoid hormones and steroids wherever possible.

Food Intolerance is a bit easier to spot – as soon as you become intolerant to a food, you will start to crave it. Watch out for any food that you start to eat every day and stop it immediately. If you start eating a particular food daily, or even more than once a day, you are right on the edge of a new intolerance so cut back before the cravings return. Be extra alert for food families (these are covered in the chapter on Food Intolerance). If you find you are eating porridge for breakfast, whole wheat salad sandwiches for lunch and whole wheat pasta for dinner and are starting to find that you are craving some or all of even these healthy foods, you could have (re)developed a Food Intolerance to wheat. Porridge, bread and pasta are all in the same food family. If you find you are quite quickly developing new cravings then try to eat foods from different food families, especially the grains. Eat rice based things one day, wheat based the next, avoid both and have potatoes for carbohydrates on the next day, and so on.

Hypoglycaemia is easier still to spot – some people get so in tune with their bodies that they know, for example, apples are fine but bananas are too sweet for them. You can't go wrong with meat, fish, Tofu, Quorn, eggs, dairy and vegetables as far as Hypoglycaemia is concerned, but as soon as you eat higher carbohydrate foods (even fruits and grains) you may find that your blood glucose level is upset. Watch out for a sudden high (energy rush) followed by a low (energy dip) as this is one of the quickest and most obvious indications that Hypoglycaemia is present.

So, here is the secret to having your cake and eating it. The guidelines for Phase 3 are:

1) Don't 'cheat' too much

2) Don't 'cheat' too often

3) Be alert and stay in control

Number 1 says don't 'cheat' too much – eat a chocolate bar if you fancy one but don't eat ten! Eat a dessert if you want one, but try to avoid processed foods in the rest of the meal. Remember your mentality will be changed so you won't think, if you eat a bag of crisps, *"I've blown the day, I may as well eat what I want."* There are no 'good' days and 'bad' days – you are in Phase 3 now, happy with your weight, so you can eat what you want **almost** when you want. You may choose to eat ice cream but you won't choose to eat a three litre tub. Number 1 is, therefore, about the **quantity** of the processed foods that you eat.

Number 2 says don't 'cheat' too often. Have a dessert for a special occasion, but just not every day.

Eat confectionery if you want to, but not every day. Have a blow out at a dinner party or a wedding but just don't do it every day. Number 2 is, therefore, about the **frequency** with which you eat processed foods. Try to stick to the rules in Phase 2 as often as possible and then cheat on special occasions, or when you really fancy something.

Number 3, as explained above, is about you having the knowledge and the skills to control your cravings and, therefore, to control your eating and your weight. Get to know what works for you like the back of your hand. You may get it wrong the first time and you may find that the cravings return strong and fast. Don't panic. Get straight back on Phase 1 for five days then Phase 2 for however long it takes to get back in control and then learn from the experience. (You may find you can just go back to Phase 2 for a few days and the cravings may subside as quickly as they arrived and you can get back in control easily).

When you learn from the experience ask yourself some questions – Were you cheating too much (quantity)? Were you cheating too often (frequency)? I bet you were more than half aware that you were starting to become quite attached to a particular food or foods and, therefore, you should have cut back earlier as this was the first sign of cravings. Be really honest with yourself next time and as soon as you think you **need** something rather than **want** something, avoid that food, like the plague, for at least five days.

Your entire goal, with eating, from now on is to stay in control of cravings. Cravings make you overeat when all you want is to be slim. You now know how to overcome the cravings. Phase 3 is about making sure that you control them, rather than that they control you, for life.

HOW long is Phase 3?

For the rest of your life. This is the way to stay at your natural weight and to eat what you want to the limit of what you can get away with. What you are really doing is following the three rules in Phase 2 but with the freedom to cheat not too much and not too often so that you stay in control of cravings for ever.

WHEN do you eat?

When you are hungry. Ideally three main meals a day with snacks in between only if you are genuinely hungry. The key point in Phase 3 is that you should limit the number of times you make your body release insulin – especially more insulin than is needed, as will happen if you cheat. So, if you really fancy a box of chocolates, you are much better off eating the whole box at once, than you are having one or two, here and there, throughout the day. If you eat a whole box of chocolates, your body won't recognise the food so it will pump out insulin to respond to the sweetness. If you eat the whole box in less than an hour, your body will have one sugar rush to respond to. If you eat the whole box throughout the day, your pancreas will be on continual alert and you will be on a roller coaster of blood glucose highs and lows for hours.

We noted earlier in the book that we have been advised to 'graze', to 'eat little and often' and to 'keep our blood glucose level constantly topped up'. As you now know, insulin is the fattening hormone and the chance of getting just the right amount released every time, to mop up whatever we have eaten, is very small. We are better off, therefore, not putting constant strain on this delicate mechanism by grazing and asking it to pump out insulin every couple of hours.

HOW much do you eat?

As much as you want but you will find some top tips for advanced cheating below.

WHY does Phase 3 work?

You overeat because of food cravings. Your goal in Phase 1 was to attack the causes of the food cravings. Your goal in Phase 2 was to eliminate the food cravings. Your goal in Phase 3 is to make sure you stay in control so that the cravings don't return. If the cravings don't return you will not be a food addict and you will be able to enjoy a bit of what you fancy when you fancy it.

Remember the goals of Phase 3:

- To put you back in control of your eating by giving you long term control over food cravings.

- To enable you to eat, without cravings, for life.

- To enable you to eat whatever you want **almost** whenever you want but with you managing the outcome.

HOW will you feel?

Like a bird let out of a cage. You really can feel liberated and empowered in a way you may find difficult to imagine right now. Just think how you would feel if you could do the following and stay at your natural weight:

- Never feel hungry and know that you need never feel hungry again.

- Know that you need never go on a fad diet again or count calories or count carbohydrates or count anything.

- Have a box of Belgian chocolates for lunch one day – because you really fancy one.

- Have steak, seafood, pasta, cheese and desserts as things that you can eat regularly because you know the 'rules'.

- Have lunch out and eat tomatoes and mozzarella with olive oil for starter; a delicious creamy, cheesy dish for main course; and then strawberries and cream for dessert. And this isn't even cheating!

- Go to a dinner party, skip the bread and carbohydrates, eat any fat and protein put in front of you, indulge in a portion of the hosts' real French chocolate mousse for dessert, and have everyone wondering where you put it all.

I can give these as real examples because this is how I can now really enjoy food and stay slim, which is what has led to so many comments from friends and colleagues. (I skip the steak, however).

Psychologically, the feelings that come from true freedom from food addiction are incredible:

- Freedom from food obsession;

- Freedom to get on with your life and to hardly think about food from when you wake until when you sleep;

- Freedom to accept and enjoy social invitations and any food that may be there;

- Freedom from guilt, fear, self-loathing and feeling like a failure;

- Freedom from diets and fresh starts;

- Freedom from time wasted because all your energy and ambition is being channelled into eating or not eating;

- Freedom from hunger and overeating hangovers.

Top tips for cheating

The basics are really worth repeating – don't cheat too much, don't cheat too often and be alert and stay in control. There are, however, some other great tips that you may like to take on board to become a real cheating connoisseur.

Cheat all at once

As was advised earlier in this chapter, if you want a box of chocolates eat the box but don't eat one or two chocolates throughout the day. Remember, you are trying to minimise the number of times your pancreas is asked to release insulin.

Eat as few ingredients as possible

The fewer processed ingredients you can attack your body with the better. If you really fancy a bag of crisps/chips then have a bag, but pick the one that has the simple ingredients potatoes and vegetable oil. There are some packets of crisps/chips that have more than one hundred ingredients in them. (The ingredients in a well-known global brand of crisps/chips, for example, are: dried potatoes with citric acid, monoglycerides or sodium phosphate; vegetable oil; corn meal; wheat starch; maltodextrin; water; salt; seasoning; spices; flavouring; acetic acid; malic acid; sodium acetate; sodium citrate; mono and diglycerides and dextrose). Please don't ever be that nasty to your body.

If you want ice cream then have Haagen-Dazs vanilla, which has (in order) fresh cream, skimmed milk, sugar, egg yolk and natural vanilla flavouring and tastes as good as ice cream can possibly get. Don't pick the carton with more ingredients than you can recognise let alone remember.

Have a strategy for getting your blood glucose level back to normal

If you eat a processed food, your body will almost certainly release too much insulin and this will make your blood glucose level fall below what it was before you ate the substance. Your body will then demand food to get your blood glucose level back to normal. This is the time when you are most at risk of craving another processed food. So, anticipate that this will happen and have something healthy to hand when you feel your blood glucose level drop. This can be a piece of fruit or a wholemeal cereal bar – any whole food that will encourage your blood glucose level to return to normal naturally.

Don't eat your normal meal AND cheat

If you are going to have a box of chocolates for lunch then make that your lunch. Don't have your steak and salad as well, as your body will just store the fat in the steak when you eat carbohydrates.

Don't waste cheating

If you are going out for dinner with friends don't start on the crisps and nuts before dinner – you know you'll eat them all as soon as you start so don't even have one. Save the indulgence for the lovely food your hosts have prepared and eat what you really want during the meal. Ditto, when eating out in restaurants don't eat the white bread at the start of the meal and fill yourself up on something that isn't even that tasty. Save your cheating for the real food and enjoy something really special from the menu instead.

Never forget that insulin is the fattening hormone

Carbohydrates stimulate the production of insulin, the fattening hormone, but so does caffeine. You may like to return to full caffeine coffee and (diet) cola in Phase 3 but this must be counted as cheating. Every time you have caffeine, you stimulate the production of insulin. If this is really how you want to use your cheating then do so. (I prefer chocolate myself). Cheating connoisseurs never forget that the key to cheating is to minimise the production of insulin.

Get to know your body

Really get to know your body, exactly what you want, how much you can get away with and how you will feel when you do cheat. Make informed choices and if a clear head and a great night's sleep are more important to you than a sugar induced stupor then make the best choice for you. If you want that sugar, however, then …

Have what you want, what you really, really want

To misquote the Spice Girls, if you want chocolate, get the best that you can find and afford. Don't settle for a confectionery bar bought from the petrol/gas station, which is more sugar than chocolate. Buy some Belgian chocolates and indulge. Keep them all to yourself, enjoy every one and feel the joy of eating something knowing you are in control of your eating.

Just because you can cheat doesn't mean you have to

This diet lets you eat all the foods that are healthy and nutritious – fruits, salads, vegetables, whole grains, animal and vegetable protein. You will not miss out on anything by not eating processed foods again so, if you don't have any urge to 'cheat', then don't.

The Harcombe Diet – A Summary

PHASE 1 – 5 DAYS

- **Do eat** meat, fish, eggs, (Tofu – if you are tolerant to soy products), Natural Live Yoghurt, any salads, any vegetables (except potatoes or mushrooms), some brown rice, herbs and spices, olive oil and butter.

- **Do drink** still or sparkling water, herbal teas, decaffeinated tea or coffee.

- **Don't eat** anything that is not on the list above. No fruit, no wheat or grains (other than brown rice) no white rice, no sugar, no cakes, no biscuits, no confectionery, no cheese, no pickled or processed foods.

- **Don't drink** alcohol, fruit juices, soft drinks, low calorie soft drinks, caffeinated products or milk.

PHASE 2 – WHILE YOU NEED TO LOSE WEIGHT

- **Rule 1** – Don't eat processed foods.

- **Rule 2** – Don't eat fats and carbohydrates at the same meal.

- **Rule 3** – Don't eat foods that cause **your** cravings.

PHASE 3 – LIFE-LONG

- Don't cheat too much.

- Don't cheat too often.

- Be alert and stay in control.

TOP VITAMIN AND MINERALS TIP

- Take a multi vitamin and mineral tablet daily, as an 'insurance policy'.

Part 5
Psychological Factors

Part 5

An Introduction

There are numerous books available saying that overeating and food addiction are purely **psychological** issues. I don't know of any books, before this one, that have fully explained the **physical** reasons for overeating: How calorie counting alone can turn a healthy person into an obsessed 'foodie'. How Candida, Food Intolerance and Hypoglycaemia can create addict-like cravings for everyday foods.

You know by now, therefore, that I'm not going to suggest that you overeat because "*Fat is a feminist Issue*", or anything like that. I fundamentally believe that you overeat because of some very common physical conditions and you need to overcome these to have a healthy relationship with food.

There are, however, some interesting psychological aspects of eating and overeating and this section of the book goes into a number of these relevant areas to do with the psychology of eating, overeating and eating disorders.

In Chapter 9, I will share my own personal experience and how I came to write this book. I really hope that sharing how my physical problems were addressed psychologically by the medical profession will help you.

In the following chapter we will look at eating disorders in general and the 'good day' and 'bad day' syndrome, in which so many people find themselves.

Chapter 11 presents the argument that we overeat because of physical reasons. There may be psychological things going on, but 1.1 billion overweight people don't all have a psychological reason for overeating. The 'developed' world has created this number of food addicts with the terrible diet advice it has given out for decades.

Finally – Chapter 12 has some helpful tips on positive thinking – to give you the tool kit to fight those unhelpful thoughts that pop into your head. *"Oh go on, it won't hurt..."* You know the ones I mean.

9

Eating Disorders – Mine

My Personal Story

I have had two phobias in my life. The first I only ever had to confront once, in a bar in Thailand of all places, but the second I had to confront every hour of every day for approximately 12 years. The first phobia was snakes. The second was food. Thankfully, I have cured myself of both.

I was the only daughter of parents who had grown up with food rationing during the war. My brother, Adrian, and I were encouraged, as a result, to eat everything put in front of us. Adrian had no problem with this, but I started a series of constant battles as I refused to eat foods that I didn't like. The conflict went on at primary school as well as at home and it was no surprise therefore that, when I reached 15, the first thing I tried to take control of was my eating.

At 15, and weighing a healthy eight and a half stone for my 5ft 2in height, I bought a book about calorie counting. This was the biggest mistake I ever made. Before long I knew the calories in every food in the supermarket, years before food labelling gave a helping hand. I cut back to 1000 calories per day, as the book advised, and the weight fell off. I now know that this is what happens with the first calorie controlled diet but the long-term problems caused by that first diet are considerable.

As my weight dropped below seven stone, my periods stopped and fine hair grew all over my body as it tried to keep me warm. I was freezing, even on a midsummer's day, and continually exhausted, but stepping on the scales and seeing further weight loss more than made up for this. At my lowest weight I was six stone and no longer a healthy teenager. My curvy figure had totally disappeared, my friends and parents were worried sick and the teachers had never seen anything like it.

I bizarrely have quite fond memories of my time as an anorexic. Anorexia is more about control than food (I was trying to regain the control that the adults had tried to take away by force feeding me) and boy did I feel in control. The self-denial felt fantastic. I was proud of my willpower and my jutting collarbones and I felt really strong. What I didn't anticipate was what would happen next...

My period of control ended almost as soon as I reached 6st and I found myself craving food like a drug addict. I entered a horrific period of approximately 10 years of bingeing and starving – one form of bulimia.

Whilst anorexia feels good and virtuous, bulimia is the exact opposite. The self-loathing that accompanies bulimia knows no boundaries. I literally hated myself and the body I was in. I never went over about 9st 7lb, but this was still more than a 50% increase on my lowest weight and to me this was quite unbearable. I never 'self harmed', but some bulimics do because they literally want to destroy their own body. Indeed, anorexia has been called 'the slow suicide'.

The mental equivalent of 'self harm' is 'beating oneself up' and I certainly did that. I would instruct myself only to have fruit one day, or just 300 calories another day, and then I would feel dreadfully guilty if I had one apple over 'my allowance'. I would never have treated my worst enemy in this way and yet I did it to myself day after day.

It is difficult to explain to someone, who has never suffered anorexia or bulimia, what it is like to be terrified of food. Think of any phobia that you may have – snakes, spiders, speaking in public – and then think what it would be like to have to face that phobia several times a day and to know that you would die without it.

People with eating disorders need to eat but they fear food, weight and calories with a quite obsessive mentality. Imagine being both obsessed with, and yet terrified of, food.

My most vivid memories of bulimia are of self-inflicted isolation. I was terrified of social situations, as I would not be able to control the food on offer. I would decline many invitations on this basis and then, invariably, I would binge throughout the time I was due to be at the event out of sheer loneliness and emptiness.

Days were either 'good' (eat hardly anything) or 'bad' (eat everything you could lay your hands on). There never seemed to be anything in between. The longest I ever went without any food at all was four days. The most I ever binged on was probably a week's 'calorie allowance' in one day – whole gourmet ice cream gateaux's, multi packs of crisps, boxes of chocolates, chips smothered in ketchup – all processed foods that did little to satisfy my insatiable cravings. Some nights I would be so hungry I couldn't fall asleep and other nights so stuffed that I struggled to wake up.

Every day that I did wake up I would vow to make a fresh start and continue to be utterly demoralised by failure. It felt like a nightmare that would never end.

The one question that kept coming into my head was – why am I doing this? I spent far too much of my precious time at Cambridge University shut away in my room stuffing my face, or avoiding fabulous social events, because I couldn't bear to attend a dinner. I kept thinking – I'm a bright girl – what on earth am I doing this for?!

Discovering the three conditions

It took almost a decade – throughout my 20's – before I could answer that question. During my time at Cambridge, I was suffering all three of the conditions and this is why I was craving food like a drug addict and why I just couldn't stick to a diet, or stop eating.

The first condition was diagnosed while I was at Cambridge and I was very lucky to be treated by one of the UK's specialists in the field of **Food Intolerance**. A very forward thinking doctor had read something about Food Intolerance and also thought it was a bit strange that I was craving food so strongly and having such strange symptoms after eating certain foods, not all food. Under the supervision of the renowned Dr Brostoff, I made huge progress, but I had only found the first piece in the jigsaw.

The second condition was diagnosed in my early to mid 20's, as I literally passed out on the tube on the way into work some mornings. This was **Hypoglycaemia**. A not so forward thinking doctor said, whenever I felt that my blood glucose level was low I should just eat a Mars Bar®! I now know this would have sent me into a roller coaster of high and low blood glucose level and this doctor should have known better.

The third condition completed the jigsaw and this was diagnosed and treated by a nutritionist when I was in my late 20's – **Candida**.

Only when I had all the pieces of the jigsaw could I understand the whole picture of why people crave food insatiably and why people can't stick to diets.

I have experienced and researched all three conditions and they all, together, explain overeating. The first diagnosis, Food Intolerance, helped me understand cravings for very particular foods – bread, cakes and cereal mainly – all from the wheat family.

When I stopped eating wheat, I increased my intake of what I thought was healthy food and I ate loads of fruit. This caused my blood glucose level to fluctuate every time I had fruit and I would eat fruit in large quantities – thinking it to be good for me. I also followed the advice to eat little and often – what bad advice this is. Knowing that insulin is the fattening hormone – why would anyone want to eat in such a way as to encourage insulin to be released every couple of hours?! This was where my Hypoglycaemia was born. With a diabetic brother, the chances were I was always going to have a more sensitive blood glucose level system than the average person and eating so many carbohydrates, even fruit, was a really bad idea.

The fruit also fed Candida beautifully. Even when I knew about Food Intolerance and Hypoglycaemia, I still craved mushrooms and vinegar in salad dressings. I also had immense cravings for bread and sweets – even though I knew from my knowledge of Food Intolerance that I shouldn't be eating either of them. The cravings were just the most awful thing imaginable. I wanted to eat sensibly. I wanted to be slim, but the desire to eat certain foods was so great, it overcame even my enormous desire to be slim. This is where the book *Why do you overeat? When all you want is to be slim* came from.

The most wonderful emails I get are from readers who have managed to overcome their own food addiction and they are now living free from cravings in a way they couldn't have believed. One woman said "*I just wish I'd known this 10 years ago*" and boy could I relate to that comment. If only I had known at University what I know now, so much time could have been better spent.

What I learned from my experience

I now know that anorexia only has two endings – the sufferer will die or they will eat more. It really is a stark as that. Horrifically 20% of sufferers die from the disease – anorexia has the highest death rate of any 'mental' illness. Those who don't die will inevitably end up eating more and, almost without exception, they will end up bingeing on food and developing food addiction, overeating and, often, bulimia.

I also know that this is no coincidence. The starvation and deprivation experienced by anorexics directly causes the subsequent overeating, for those who survive the disease.

Anorexia is just the most extreme example of everything outlined in this book. The anorexic has the direct outcomes from eating so little – getting hungry; losing lean muscle and storing fat and slowing their metabolisms down. They will eat mostly carbohydrates, what little they do eat. They will eat the same foods every day – almost ritually and they will have horribly weakened their immune systems. They will then also have all the indirect outcomes of eating less. I would be astonished if every anorexic does not have Candida, Food Intolerance and/or Hypoglycaemia.

The average calorie counter is doing exactly the same as an anorexic – just to a less extreme extent. The calorie counter will still get hungry, lose lean muscle, slow their metabolism down and get the three conditions that cause food cravings. The most important thing I learned from my experience was never to count calories again.

How the personal story ends

The story has a very happy ending as I have been totally free from eating problems for over 12 years and have easily maintained a healthy weight of eight stone throughout this time. The weight maintenance phase

(Phase 3) is the fun part of the book, as this is where I have been for over a decade.

I could have written this book 10 years ago but it wasn't until my friends and colleagues got fed up with me being able to eat so much without putting on weight that they badgered me into sharing the secret. The secret of Phase 3 is not to cheat too much or too often and to make sure that the conditions that cause cravings never return. You will be stunned at how easy this is once your immune system is back in good shape and you stop starving your body of the energy that it needs.

I have not feared food in any way for years. I love it. I eat huge portions and never suffer from bloating or discomfort, as used to happen after eating food. I love porridge, berries and cream, cappuccinos, pasta, cheese and anything my husband cooks for me. My favourite food of all is chocolate. I don't mean confectionery, but anything with at least 70%+ cocoa content. I am a member of a chocolate tasting club and I enjoy chocolate like many people enjoy wine. I am the first to accept any dinner or lunch invitation – I love eating out and can't wait to see what will be put in front of me. I will never again turn down a social event because of food – on the contrary I will accept an invite because I hope the food will be fantastic.

With the exception of "*The Happy Ending*" bit, I struggled to write this part of the book. The only way I can understand my years with an eating disorder (first anorexia and then bulimia) is to look back at the notes that I made at the time. I don't know the person who wrote those notes. I really find it difficult to imagine how she felt because the person who wrote those notes just isn't me any more. I am so pleased to be able to say that I have moved on so far and left that whole nightmare behind.

The statistics on the incidence of eating disorders means that you are likely to know someone just like the person that I was. They may well be your child, partner, relative, colleague, friend, or this article may be talking to you personally. My heart goes out to you because I genuinely can say – even though the memories have faded – I know how you feel.

10

Eating Disorders – Generally

Types of eating disorder

There are three main types of eating disorder – anorexia, bulimia and compulsive eating.

The medical definition of anorexia is "*loss of appetite*" but this is a really ironic definition of anorexia as an eating disorder. Anorexia (real loss of appetite) can follow from a traumatic incident, like the loss of a loved one. Anorexia, as an eating disorder, is quite deliberate abstention from eating despite probable ravenous hunger. It is a conscious decision, not a subconscious reaction to a traumatic incident. It results in a sudden, rapid weight loss leading to an abnormally low body weight. Women suffering from anorexia often find that their periods stop. The sufferer will feel continually cold even in warm weather and 'down-like' hair may grow all over the body, as nature tries to make up for the lost heat energy. Mentally, anorexia is characterised by a paranoid fear of food and of putting on weight. Interest in food, calories, weight and size is obsessive and the single minded determination to avoid food can make a normally honest person secretive and dishonest, as the anorexic will do anything to avoid eating.

This book is not really for anorexics because we are trying to understand overeating, not the opposite. However, this book may be able to help anorexics in three ways:

1) Many anorexics have periods of uncontrolled eating as part of their disorder and this book can help explain why they crave food (especially particular foods);

2) Anorexia often comes before bulimia or compulsive eating, so the anorexic should use this book to learn

about what is likely to happen if they continue to try to live on so few calories. The anorexic's continuous starvation is laying the foundations for Candida, Food Intolerance and Hypoglycaemia.

3) The Harcombe Diet helps people reach their natural weight. Any anorexic, whose survival instinct wins through, will be able to reach their natural weight following the advice in this book. They do not need to be 'force fed' calories in hospital wards. Eating real food, not processed calories, and teaching the anorexic finally to nourish and nurture herself (or himself) is the best way of giving the anorexic back their self-worth.

The general point to make here, in this chapter on psychological factors, is that anorexia does seem to have psychological roots. Various authors have discussed these at length and I'm not planning to go into them any further here. As shared in "*My Personal Story*", my own anorexia started as a desire to gain control in some way over my life and this is still the single most common factor behind anorexia. Whenever I hear the word anorexia, I think control, as this is what anorexia is really about.

Anorexia is of more interest to us as an extreme example of how calorie deprivation leads to Candida, Food Intolerance and Hypoglycaemia and how there are physical foundations underlying binge eating disorders.

From the one eating disorder that is about under-eating, we turn to the two that are about overeating – bulimia and compulsive eating. The distinction between the two is generally assumed to be that bulimics overeat and then attempt to compensate by taking laxatives and/or being sick and/or starving, whilst compulsive eaters overeat without necessarily trying to purge or starve afterwards.

What are the symptoms?

Physically, bulimics tend to be normal or near normal weight whilst compulsive eaters may be considerably overweight. However, as a result of their attempts to purge their binges, bulimics may suffer from other physical symptoms – tiredness, stomach problems, dry skin and hair, muscle weakness, headaches, palpitations and tooth decay to name just a few of the many side effects. Bulimic women can also find that their periods stop. Vitamin and mineral deficiency inevitably occurs, as the absorption of food is disturbed.

Psychologically there is little to distinguish bulimics and compulsive eaters from anorexics – all share the same paranoid fear of food and of putting on weight and a complete obsession with food. All overeaters, whether lapsed anorexics, bulimics or compulsive eaters, would identify with some or all of the following descriptions of themselves:

- To be obsessed with, yet terrified of, food.

- To think about food from the minute you wake up until the minute you fall asleep.

- To be terrified of putting on weight.

- To fear social situations where you may not be able to determine what food may be on offer.

- To decline social invitations for this reason.

- To decline social invitations because you want to lose weight before seeing so-and-so again.

- To judge a day purely by the amount of food you have, or have not, consumed, not by what you have done or achieved.

- To be overwhelmed with guilt for eating an apple if you vowed not to eat an apple that day.

- To hate yourself.

- To feel a failure.

- To decline a dinner invitation as you don't intend to eat that day.

- To decline a dinner invitation for the above reason and then stuff yourself for the entire evening instead.

- To make a fresh start each and every day.

- To be utterly demoralised by continuous failure.

- To lose all faith and confidence in yourself.

- To feel that you are having a nightmare that will never end.

- To waste vast amounts of potential because all your energy and ambition is being channelled into eating or not eating.

- To be unable to sleep some nights due to genuine hunger.

- To collapse into a heavy sleep after a binge and to wake the next morning puffy eyed, bloated, hungover and fat.

- To have two wardrobes.

- To not be able to plan ahead because you don't know what weight you will be and hence you won't know if you will even want to attend a social occasion let alone what you will wear.

- To continually set yourself tougher and tougher 'rules' in an attempt to control your behaviour.

- To feel totally out of control nonetheless.

- To hate the lies and deception, which accompany food addiction as, you try to avoid food or social occasions.

- To want to be open but to feel the world will despise you.

- To put off living until tomorrow "*when I'll be slim.*"

- To exist not to live.

If you empathise with any, or all, of the above statements this book can help you find a way out from this. The above list describes a nightmare – the most horrible place to be. I wrote the above list back in the 1980s when my eating was out of control. I read the list now and struggle to empathise with it at all, but I am so glad that I kept the notes I wrote then to remind me of a place I never want to return to.

To be a healthy, slim person living inside a fat body is literally to feel that you cannot live with yourself. You want to escape your body and leave the fat that you loathe so much behind. The pain and despair faced by food addicts knows no limits. But there is a way out. There is a way to stop the food addiction and to stop the overeating. This is what The Harcombe Diet is about.

Good days and bad days

There is a current epidemic of overeating. Millions of people in the developed world are waking each morning wondering whether the day will be 'good' or 'bad'. We are not thinking about the weather, or about what we will do at work or leisure. We are thinking about what and how much we will eat.

On a 'good' day we will get through the time from when we get up to when we go to bed without overeating. The relevant words here are 'get through'. The day is never easy. It is a complete effort of willpower, a continuous struggle against the urge to eat. Some people will go to great lengths to avoid temptation – even to the extent of staying in bed or taking a trip into the countryside away from shops. In the UK, in the 1980s, there was a tragic story, which made national headlines, about a bulimic aerobics teacher who faked her own disappearance one December rather than face all the overeating opportunities that Christmas gives. How many of us understood her extreme measures. Any reader familiar with the 'good' day scenario will know that it ends with a sense of achievement, but also an underlying fear that the period of being in control with food is likely to be short-lived. This is usually the case.

On a 'bad' day we will not be able to resist the urge to eat and, having started, we may not be able to stop. Many overeaters eat so fast that they do not taste the food. Most rarely enjoy much more than the first mouthful, if that. Many eat way beyond the feeling of fullness. Many continue to eat even when they feel bloated or even physically sick.

Yet we want more than anything else to be slim. Magazines ask which we would rather happen: to be and stay at our ideal weight for life; to win the lottery; to meet the partner of our dreams; or to land our dream job. Guess what comes top? How can we question the desire to be slim? It is at the top, heading the list, of the most desirable things in the world.

People are prepared to take tablets to slim or even contemplate stomach stapling or jaw wiring – how much does this tell you about their desire to be slim? And yet more of us than ever are overweight and the numbers are rising at an alarming rate. The one conclusion you have to reach is that what we are currently doing doesn't work. Counting calories, fad diets, slimming pills are clearly not the answer or obesity would not be an issue let alone an epidemic. Why, why, why, therefore, do we overeat?

11

Why Do We Overeat?

I think that the psychological reasons for overeating have a part to play, but they have been given way too much importance in the overall explanation. Sure, we eat when we are lonely or bored or depressed etc. but this doesn't explain why we crave food like drug addicts.

I remember being referred to an eating disorder specialist when I had my problems in my 20's. I remember being asked endless questions about my relationship with my mother and my views on my sexuality (did I not like the attention my curves got from men – that kind of thing). And all I could think about was wading my way through a box of chocolates. To me, this wasn't about just generally overeating, but wanting to eat very specific things. If I was using food in some emotional way – how come I only wanted to eat processed foods? How come I never craved salmon and green beans? Why did I like to eat salad, but only if it had salad dressing on it? (I now know that I was craving the vinegar to 'feed' Candida).

The psychological reasons behind overeating have a place in the theory of the condition, but they are not sufficient as explanations. There is a lot going on psychologically when we overeat, but far more important is what is going on physically. The willpower needed by overeaters to resist the urge to binge is so intense that it cannot be less than the desire an alcoholic has for a drink or a smoker has for a cigarette. Yet overeaters are treated as people with no willpower, at best, or a psychological condition at worst. Why are alcoholics and smokers treated as addicts with a physical problem (and possible secondary emotional problems) when overeaters are seen as people with a psychological disorder? Why are overeaters also not seen as addicts just like alcoholics or drug addicts?

I get so mad when I get emails from people who have been called "*greedy*" or "*weak-willed*" by their doctors or dieticians. I also get so frustrated when I hear doctors and dieticians say they just can't understand why their patients can't stick to a diet – "*what is wrong with them*?" they say.

I believe that, if someone wants to be slim as badly as most people I know, then, if they overeat, it is because something else is going on. I have huge faith in people and their commitment to achieve something that they really want. So, if someone really wants to be slim, and they find themselves eating a packet of biscuits, that honestly, they do not want to be eating, that is not greed. That is an addiction, so strong, that it is even greater than their desire to be slim.

People overeat because they are food addicts. Your cravings for food, which drive you to overeat, are as strong as those cravings experienced by drink or drug addicts. At the exact moment you overeat, your desire to eat is stronger than even your immense desire to be slim. You do desperately want to be slim. You wake up determined, you stick to a diet for a couple of hours or days but then you have a craving so overwhelming that you will drive to a 7-11 in the middle of the night or you will eat the children's sweets or you will possibly even take things out of the dustbin that you threw away yesterday to stop you eating them. You are not a failure. You are not greedy or weak-willed. This is not your fault. You are addicted to food. You can, however, change this.

This book is, therefore, very relevant to the bulimic or compulsive eater – to anyone who overeats regardless of whether or not they try to purge the binge. This book is saying that whilst psychological factors do have an important part to play in the understanding of eating disorders, there are physical reasons why people overeat which are just as important if not more so.

The physical reasons are (you should know them off by heart by now):

- Calorie counting, which will make anyone with an eating disorder hungry and likely to crave food.

- Candida, which will make sufferers crave yeasty, sugary, vinegar foods.

- Food Intolerance, which will make sufferers crave specific foods or food families.

- Hypoglycaemia, which will make sufferers crave carbohydrates.

Given the abuse anorexics, bulimics and compulsive eaters have given their bodies, they are extremely likely to be candidates for all three of the conditions in this book. Their immune systems will not be in a good state. They will have depleted their bodies of nutrients for some time and they will be very susceptible to Candida, Food Intolerance and Hypoglycaemia.

Anyone with a serious eating disorder, like anorexia or bulimia, should work through this book, like any other person prone to overeating, as the reasons for the overeating and the conditions being suffered are the same.

Remember, if you overeat, you are not greedy or weak-willed. You are an addict just like a smoker or drug addict and you now have the tool kit to cure your food addiction and to stop the cravings for ever.

Eating disorders are laying the body wide open to all of the conditions of Candida, Food Intolerance and Hypoglycaemia. Eating disorders directly and indirectly cause food cravings and the best thing that you can do is to follow the advice in this book. Start being nice to your body and get the cravings well under control.

Food Addiction

Addiction to a substance has four main characteristics:

1) An uncontrollable craving;

2) Increasing tolerance, so that more of the addictive substance is needed in order to produce the same effects;

3) Physical or psychological dependence – the substance produces a feeling of wellbeing (euphoria in the extreme) when you first consume it and then, in the latter stages of the addiction, the substance is needed to avoid unpleasant withdrawal feelings;

4) Adverse effects on the consumer.

Food addicts will relate to the above – let us look at the four characteristics of addiction in relation to chocolate, as an example:

1) 'Chocoholics' will describe cravings for chocolate that are addict-like and quite uncontrollable;

2) The chocolate binges get worse and worse and 'chocoholics' feel the need to consume ever-increasing quantities of chocolate to satisfy their addiction;

3) The third characteristic – physical or psychological dependence – describes the situation where the addict stops getting good feelings when they eat chocolate. They actually get to the point where they need chocolate to stop the withdrawal symptoms, i.e. they need chocolate not to feel good but to stop feeling bad;

4) Finally, think about the adverse effects – the unbearable cravings, the dopey feelings, headaches, bloating, weight gain/fluctuations, water retention,

fatigue and so on. If it were not for these you would have little reason to confront the problem – you would just carry on eating chocolate. But food addiction gets worse, not better, and at some stage the adverse effects get so bad that you have to act.

In the above respects food addiction is exactly the same as alcoholism or drug addiction. Drug addicts get a fantastic high when they first take, say, heroin. Then, perhaps for a few occasions whilst taking the substance, they experience great highs. Very quickly, more quickly with some people than others, the highs wear off and the drug is then needed not to get high but to avoid the low, which becomes more and more unbearable. The craving for heroin becomes insatiable and more and more of the substance is needed to continually avoid the terror of the withdrawal symptoms. The adverse effects on the consumer at this stage are dreadful – tracks on the arms, tremors, sweats, severe weight loss, no energy, no life let alone zest for life, pale skin, shattered immune system, infections and possibly even HIV if needles have been shared.

Food addiction differs from drug addiction only in the extreme lengths people will go to for their fix and perhaps in the strength of the adverse effects. In general, drug addiction leads to more physical and mental damage than food addiction. However, if you have seen a 200-300lb person with no energy, or health, or desire for life, existing day to day rather than living, you may wonder that there is little difference in the effect that food, or heroin, can have on our wellbeing.

So how do we overcome this? What does food addiction tell us about why we are overeating? The message for overcoming overeating is this – you will continue to overeat, that is to crave food uncontrollably, unless you identify and avoid all foods to which you are addicted.

You overeat and binge compulsively because you have one, or all, of a number of conditions, which we focus on at length in Part 3 of the book. These conditions are Candida, Food Intolerance and Hypoglycaemia. You may have one, or all, of these conditions and any, or all, of them will lead to addict-like cravings. You are not weak-willed. You are not greedy. You have a health problem, or a number of health problems, and you must think of yourself like a Diabetic in that there are certain foods that you simply must avoid for your health. You are an alcoholic with food in place of alcohol. You are a nicotine addict with food in place of cigarettes.

Having compared food addiction to drink or drug addiction, there is a key factor which makes the treatment of an eating problem far more difficult than that of a drink or drug addiction. The problem is this – an alcoholic is advised to go 'cold turkey' (to totally avoid drink) just as a smoker has to totally avoid cigarettes. Indeed reformed alcoholics stick tightly to the principle 'one day at a time' and they think just one taste of alcohol could set them back on the downhill path to alcoholism. The problem for the food addict is that they cannot go 'cold turkey' (excuse the pun) on food. Overeaters have to eat but not binge. That is like telling a drug addict to have some heroin each day but not too much. A sure recipe for disaster.

Many overeaters would agree that it is easier to ban food totally than it is to eat it in moderation. The continued success of liquid diets since the 1980s supports this – many overeaters find it easier to survive on fewer than 500 calories a day, all in liquid form, than to eat real food in a calorie counted diet.

The current advice on overeating seems to be to eat everything in moderation. Many slimming clubs tell us we can eat anything, but we have to count the points allocated to each food (another way of counting calories). With calorie counting, we are told we can eat anything so long as we don't exceed a certain number of calories a day. We are told that no food is a sin, no food is bad for us and if we ban foods we will simply crave them. Why don't we advise the alcoholic to have a glass of wine, but not a whole bottle of either? Why don't we say to the smoker don't give up cigarettes or you will only crave them? This advice would be simply crazy for drink or drug addicts so how, therefore, can it possibly work for the overeater?

The fundamental problem is that food addiction is not seen as a similar problem to any other addiction. It is widely accepted that drugs, alcohol and cigarettes are addictive but it is less widely accepted that food can be addictive (although caffeine is being increasingly recognised as an addictive substance). However, in many ways, your problem is worse. An alcoholic can overcome their problem by avoiding alcohol altogether. A nicotine addict must give up cigarettes. A drug addict must stop taking drugs. You, a food addict, cannot stop eating. You have to learn to live with food and to eat in such a way that you don't overeat and, most importantly, that you don't have an uncontrollable desire to overeat. Fortunately, there is a way to do this...

You don't stop eating, but you do stop eating the foods that contribute to the conditions that are causing your cravings. This book will help you identify the conditions you may be suffering from and the foods you, therefore, need to avoid. The good news is that having a weakened immune system causes many of the conditions and they further weaken the immune system, in a vicious circle, once they take hold. So, if you can break out of the vicious circle and start improving your immune system you will be able to re-introduce foods in the future which are currently causing you problems. You must stop eating the foods that are making you overeat and overweight **now,** but you won't have to give them up for ever.

There are numerous books about Candida, Food Intolerance and Hypoglycaemia. These books all identify specific food cravings as key signs of Candida, Food Intolerance and Hypoglycaemia. Yet such information remains exclusive to books on these conditions and is rarely found in books on eating disorders. Why? We are led to believe that eating disorders are psychological disorders and not physical disorders. However, the medical evidence for food cravings, in relation to Candida, Food Intolerance and Hypoglycaemia, seems indisputable and the overeater can benefit so much from being aware of the physical factors that may be causing their irrational behaviour.

There are psychological reasons that lead people to become dependent on food. Food does act as a comfort, a stress release, and an escape. Food is like alcohol to many overeaters – when we binge we are so 'spaced out' we may as well be drunk – this may be our way of coping with the world. We do need to be aware of, and deal with, any psychological factors that may be playing a part in our overeating. However, much stronger than this, there are physical reasons why we overeat.

The essence of this book is that you will continue to overeat, to crave food uncontrollably, unless you identify and avoid all foods to which you are addicted. Cravings will be out of your control for as long as you have Candida, Food Intolerance and/or Hypoglycaemia, which are out of control.

12

How to overcome the diet destroying voices in your head

This is the most important chapter in this book. There is only one person in the world that can make sure you control your eating and that is you. I sincerely hope that this book helps to show you how but, at the end of the day, it is up to you whether or not you choose to do anything about your eating and your weight.

For as long as you are addicted to food, I firmly believe that you do not have a free choice about when and what you eat. The fact that at the particular moment that you eat the substance you do want it more than you want to be slim is a fantastic demonstration of just how powerful food addiction is.

The goal of this book is, therefore, to enable you to be free from food addiction. When you follow the advice in this book, you **will** get to the point that you are not craving food in general or specific foods. You **will** be free from food addiction and the overwhelming cravings for food that have been sabotaging your eating goals will be gone. This is when it really will be **up to you**!

At this time, when the addiction has gone, you **will** have a choice. You will not have compulsive cravings and you will be free to choose what you eat and when. At this time you need to exercise your freedom to choose on a regular basis. When you are not compulsively craving chocolate, for example, you will have an opportunity to buy chocolate (at any one of hundreds of thousands of retail outlets across the world). You will be able to make a balanced, level headed choice that you will not feel able to make right now. You will be able to weigh up how much you want the chocolate (note the word 'want' not 'need') and what it will do to you if you do have it.

The two voices that slimmers have in their head

You know what this bit is about – you want to eat but you want to be slim. You want that cream cake but you want to get into that outfit for the special occasion. We seem to have two voices going on in our heads all the time – the devil and the angel – and, depending on which one wins, we are 'bad' or 'good'.

This section is about how you silence the devil in your head and let the angel win through every time. When you start Phase 1 the devil is going to go wild. It is going to do whatever it can to get you to feed your food addiction. The Candida will physically be crying out to be fed, your Food Intolerance withdrawal symptoms will be begging you to eat your favourite substance and your Hypoglycaemia will be craving processed carbohydrates. As if these physical things are not bad enough, psychologically, you will be telling yourself the following:

1) Start tomorrow – just enjoy that pizza, chocolate, sandwich today – I can be good tomorrow.

2) A slice of pizza, one chocolate bar, one biscuit can't hurt.

3) I deserve it.

4) I feel fine – maybe I don't have all these Candida things after all.

5) I really want that chocolate bar, muffin, tub of ice cream.

6) I'm going to a dinner party tonight – it would be rude not to eat whatever is put in front of me.

7) It shouldn't go to waste (food in the house, children's leftovers etc).

8) I'm on holiday or I'm in a restaurant – I won't get the chance to eat all of this lovely stuff tomorrow.

9) I've eaten something I shouldn't have, so I'll eat what I want today and then start again tomorrow

10) Why not?!

These and more are definitely going to be in your mind when you start the diet so you need to be armed with strategies to overcome them. Here are some suggestions:

1) *Start tomorrow – just enjoy that pizza, chocolate, sandwich today – I can be good tomorrow.*

Every diet starts tomorrow. It is a cliché that tomorrow never comes but clichés are generally true. Every time you say you will start tomorrow you are doing two things:

a) You are putting off the day you take control of your eating and, therefore, your life. You are putting off living, rather than existing. You are letting your addiction rule you, rather than ruling your addiction.

b) More seriously you are making it even harder to take control with every day that you continue to be ruled by food. Food addiction does not reach a certain level and then plateau. It gets worse and worse the more you feed your addiction. Remember the characteristics of addiction – you need to consume more and more to have the same high and before long you need to consume more and more just to avoid the low – the highs are no longer there. With every day that you delay tackling food addiction it just gets worse. Yes you can start tomorrow – but it will be even tougher to crack tomorrow. **You have to do this sometime so do it now.**

2) *A slice of pizza, one chocolate bar, one biscuit can't do any harm.*

In Phase 1, any and all of the above will do harm. They are all processed carbohydrates and they will all feed your addiction. If you give in on day one you are back to square one. If you give in on day two you have wasted nearly two days – why do it? If you give in on day three you have wasted nearly three days – that's daft. Giving in on day four or five is even worse. Don't give in to these cravings. The whole purpose of this diet is to stop cravings because cravings make you overeat and overeating makes you fat. If you give into the cravings you will never get in the position that they can be controlled. All it takes is five days – stick with it, one day at a time and see for yourself.

Eat more of any food that is allowed if necessary to make you so full that you can't give into the cravings. Drink a glass of water every time you feel tempted to eat your favourite foods. **You have to do this sometime so do it now.**

3) *I deserve it*.

No matter how productive or tough a day you have had at work or at leisure you do deserve to be nice to yourself. Eating processed food is not, however, being nice to yourself. Giving in to yeast parasites growing inside you is not nice. Eating foods that your body cannot tolerate is not nice and throwing a brick on your pancreas/insulin mechanism is not nice. You deserve so much more than this. You deserve to live not to exist. You deserve to be free from food cravings. You deserve to be nourished and full of nutrients, not stuffed and full of empty calories. You deserve to be in control of your life not controlled by food. You deserve so many things but 'junk food' is at the bottom of the list.

4) *I feel fine – maybe I don't have all these Candida things after all*.

Now you are really scraping the barrel! The devil will tell you anything to try to get you to feed the

Candida, or to eat the foods to which you are addicted. The very fact that you want these foods so badly says that you are addicted to them. If you really can take them or leave them, then leave them.

If you are overweight, then you are overeating the wrong things. If you are overeating, despite desperately wanting to be slim, you are doing this because you are addicted to food. This is what cravings and food addiction are all about.

Be really honest with yourself – you are a food addict and you have to go cold turkey on your problem foods for at least five days before you can start to break free from your addiction.

5) *I really want that chocolate bar, muffin, tub of ice cream.*

Of course you do. You are physically craving it. You are addicted to it, so you want it as badly as a smoker wants a cigarette or an alcoholic wants a drink. You would do anything to get it, which is precisely why you must not have it. You must not give in. You need to break the addiction, otherwise you will continue to have your life ruled by food and will continue to overeat and be overweight for life. You will also continue to be dopey, bloated, exhausted and everything else that goes with food addiction. All your energy needs to be focused on not giving in to the cravings and ending the addiction.

6) *I'm going to a dinner party tonight – it would be rude not to eat whatever is put in front of me.*

If you are in Phase 1 – what are you doing going to a dinner party? You need to make these five days as easy as possible, not set yourself up to fail.

If you are in Phase 2 you should be fine going for a fat meal option. Just skip the bread and potatoes and fill up on prawn cocktail, casserole, meat, fish, vegetables and any fat/protein that is offered. Hopefully you know your hosts well enough to let them know that you are doing something positive for your weight and your health. If they are good hosts and care about you then they will be understanding and accommodating. A good host does not push dessert on someone trying to lose weight. They do everything that they can to make their guests feel comfortable and relaxed. Hosts are used to coping with Vegetarians, genuine food allergies and wheat-free diets. If you let your hosts know that you are there to see them, and any carbohydrate free food that they can offer will be a bonus, you will be fine.

In Phase 3 you have a choice – you can still decline the carbohydrates, if you choose, but you may choose to accept any wholemeal carbohydrates that are on offer. Or, you could decide to eat what you want, enjoy the freedom for the evening and then get back on track the next day. You are likely to get to a point when eating processed carbohydrates makes you feel so sluggish that you just don't want to do it anymore.

7) *It shouldn't go to waste*

If you are worried about food at home going to waste – why is stuff you might crave there? Stop buying processed foods. Get rid of all processed foods at home before you start Phase 1. Your family need to support you – they can benefit from healthier eating too. No one in your family, or any other family for that matter, needs processed carbohydrates so have wholemeal versions to hand instead.

If you are worried about the children's leftovers try to understand why. Does this come from your own childhood? Are you carrying a subconscious 'rule' that plates must be licked clean? Children, unlike adults, tend to have a natural appetite and they will stop eating as soon as they feel full. If you often get leftovers then reduce the portion sizes served. If it happens just with certain foods then let them decide how much they want of that food (if any). If it happens every now and again just throw the food away, or save it for later if it will keep. The food was supposed to be in your child's tummy by now so why should it matter throwing it away? Don't let any daft views on waste ruin your health.

8) *I'm on holiday or I'm in a restaurant – I won't get the chance to eat all of this lovely stuff tomorrow.*

You also won't have a chance to be slim tomorrow unless you start taking control of your eating today. Also – you will actually have a chance to eat all this 'lovely stuff' again. You can come back to the restaurant, or return to the same holiday resort, in the future. Food doesn't ever go away. How often have you eaten something because it was there not because you needed or even wanted it? If there is a box of chocolates, or a celebration cake, being shared out at work don't give in. You can buy and eat an entire box of chocolates or cake on your own tomorrow if you want – I bet you won't want to once the moment has passed.

Remember, in Phase 1 and 2, you are trying to get your cravings under control so that you can get back in control of your eating and reach your natural weight. You will be able to eat what you want **almost** when you want in Phase 3. You will be able to sample new foods on holiday. You will be able to indulge in a restaurant. You will be able to have cake and chocolates for celebrations, if this is what you want to do. You will be at your natural weight, your eating will be under control and you will enjoy these indulgences so much more because you will not feel guilty or loathe yourself for having them.

9) *I've eaten something I shouldn't have, so I'll eat what I want today and then start again tomorrow*

No one ever ruined a day's eating with that first mouthful. It is what you do after that first mouthful that ruins the day's eating...

- Let us imagine that you have vowed not to eat breakfast and then hunger takes over and you find yourself having a bowl of sugary cereal or,

_ You vowed not to eat chocolate and you find yourself buying a confectionery bar as you get a morning newspaper or,

_ You vowed to 'be good' all day but then you settle down to watch TV and suddenly those potato chips are calling to you from the kitchen...

Sounds familiar? So you give in to each of the events above, but this doesn't ruin the day's eating. It is what we do next that leads to a binge day. What do we say to ourselves? I've blown it today so I might as well eat what I want and then start afresh tomorrow. We can't be 'good' today so we will be 'bad' today and then 'good' tomorrow. And can you recall the relief and excitement you feel once you have made that decision? You suddenly 'allow' yourself to eat whatever you want. You may even get quite excited at the thought of what you will have. I could salivate at the mere thought of chocolate, miles away from getting my hands on it!

But all of this is our mind playing games. Who decided the good vs. bad rules in the first place? You did! Who decided not to have breakfast? (Crazy decision) You did! And it was you, again, who decided that the 'good' day was over. You have to be alert to the things going on in your head that are leading you to overeat. Remember – no one ever blew a diet with the first mouthful – it was what they decided to do next (yes decided) that blew it. **You** never blew a diet with the first mouthful – it was what **you** decided to do next that blew it.

Let's find a few ways around this thinking:

First of all you don't have 'good' days and 'bad' days any more – or rather you don't have them like you used to. A good day now is a day when you are nice to yourself and your body. A good day is when you nourish your body and feed it with vitamins and minerals and nutritious food. A bad day is when you are nasty to yourself and your body. This is any day when you binge or starve, or count calories, or try to give your body less food than it really needs.

Another idea is to introduce the concept of a weight maintenance day. In your old life you may only have had 'good' days or 'bad' days. In your old world these were days when you lost weight or days when you gained weight. Now you can have neutral days, when you don't gain or lose weight, but you continue to nourish your body and eat mostly healthy food but you have the freedom to cheat. This is exactly what Phase 3 is about. Ideally you will only do Phase 3 when you are at your natural weight, but you can have a Phase 3 day at any time.

If you do eat something you feel you 'shouldn't' have eaten, don't go back to your old style thinking and eat everything except the kitchen sink. Decide to have a Phase 3 day. You won't register lighter on the scales tomorrow but you won't have another couple of pounds to lose that you have just put on today. If you have something you feel you 'shouldn't' then start a weight maintenance/Phase 3 day – don't cheat too much and don't cheat too often. So finish your cheat and then get back on track for the rest of the day. Don't forget to manage the cravings that may come after eating processed carbohydrates and upsetting your blood glucose level. Eat some whole foods to help regulate your blood glucose after eating processed carbohydrates.

– If you have one slip up on this diet just get straight back on track. Don't beat yourself up. Don't make it worse and don't blow things out of proportion – '*I've had one small slip so it is the end of the diet.*' This is nonsense and you know it. Don't look for excuses to give up.

10) *Why not?*

Why not indeed? This is your life. The choice is yours. So often we look for a magic wand or for someone else to make the decisions for us in life. The decision to overeat or to get your eating in control is entirely within your hands. It is up to you. If you really want that chocolate brownie more than you want to be slim then eat it. It really is up to you. However, just stop for one moment before you do eat it and ask yourself why you want it so badly. You are an addict remember. You are not just choosing that chocolate brownie, therefore, you are choosing a way of life. You are choosing to continue to be a food addict, to continue your cravings and to continue to overeat. If you really do want to get to the point where food doesn't rule your life then you have to start by saying no to it now. The longer you say yes, the longer you will be addicted and the harder this will be to overcome when you eventually do tackle it (and you will have to for the sake of your health sooner or later). Why prolong the inevitable any longer? Say no to the craving now and say yes to a craving free future.

Part 6

Questions & Answers

Part 6

Questions & Answers

This section has been revised since the first edition of this book. As much of the book is in a question and answer format, we have taken out the questions covered in earlier chapters to avoid repetition.

This has enabled us to include many new questions, every one of which comes from readers of *Why do you overeat?* and/or *Stop Counting Calories*. There have been so many questions that we are now able to establish a clear Top 10 most Frequently Asked Questions (FAQ's). We hope that the following pages answer any queries that you may have:

1) The Top 10 FAQ's (sweeteners, soya milk, avocados, honey, yoghurt, hummus, sweet potatoes, nuts and seeds, tofu and Quorn);

2) The Harcombe Diet vs. traditional diet advice;

3) Candida, Food Intolerance and Hypoglycaemia – additional queries beyond those covered in Part 3;

4) Cravings;

5) Specific foods (beyond the Top 10): sugar-free gum, chips, pulses, tomatoes – if you've asked about a food, it's in here. These are in alphabetical order, but please check the index at the back of the book for your particular food query;

6) Carbs, fats, protein and mixing – clearing up any confusion;

7) Shopping;

8) Drinks;

9) Medical considerations – Constipation, Diabetes, and Pregnancy amongst others;

10) Personal Questions.

1) The Top 10 FAQ's

Q) Can I have sweeteners/sugar substitutes?

A) My advice would be **not** to eat artificial sweeteners because this book is all about a) eating healthily and b) getting rid of cravings. Let us look at each of these two points:

a) I can't see how anything artificial fits in with healthy eating. Some sweeteners have been banned. We may discover others to be harmful, in time. We can be confident that sweeteners have no positive impact on our health and that we have no physiological need for them, (because they have no nutrients – just like sugar).

b) The second key thing is that we are trying to get rid of cravings and the most common cravings are for sweet foods, whether as a result of Candida, Food Intolerance, Hypoglycaemia, or all three. If you continue to feed your body artificially sweet things, you will continue to want artificially sweet things and the cravings won't disappear.

I have also found compelling evidence in obesity journals that sweeteners have much the same impact on the body and insulin mechanism as sugar – the body can't tell the difference and so releases insulin unnecessarily.

What you can have, as an alternative to sweetener, is something called Fructooligosaccharide (FOS). This is a non-digestible, soluble-fibre carbohydrate that supports the growth of good bacteria in our guts. It passes through our intestines and is cleverly used by lactobacilli and other friendly flora to aid their growth. You can buy it in health food shops and sprinkle it on porridge, or other cereal, if you really long for something sweet. It turns into a chewy, toffee like substance in your mouth.

Q) Can I have soya milk?

A) In Phase 1, ideally no, as we are getting back to the basics of meat, fish, eggs, vegetables and salad ("MEVY"). However, if you have never craved soya milk (so there is no risk of Food Intolerance), it is not going to be that bad if you have it in Phase 1. It can be particularly useful for a Vegetarian to have soya milk for some more food options for Phase 1.

In Phase 2 – yes you can. Soya milk is naturally low fat (it is less than 2% fat, which is only slightly higher than skimmed cow's milk). Check the fat content on your particular product. If for some strange reason your version is a more concentrated version of soya milk, it may be higher than 2% in fat. If this is the case, try to find a lower fat version. If it is no more than 2-3% fat, it is absolutely fine with pure porridge oats or brown rice cereal – perfect carb breakfasts.

Q) Can I eat avocados?

A) In Phase 1, no, because an avocado is a fruit.

In Phase 2, in a 100g portion of avocado, there are 15g of fat and 9g of carbohydrate. Avocados are, therefore, higher in fat than carbs, but have quite high levels of both. This means you should eat them in moderation in Phase 2 and have them as part of a fat meal on the occasions when you do have them.

In Phase 3, cheat with them as much as you want.

Q) Is honey OK?

A) Honey is a more natural product than sugar and it has some (small) nutritional value, so I'm less anti-honey than I am anti-sugar. However, it is still a processed product and it is 100% carbohydrate – it doesn't even contain protein. In this respect it is in the same league as sugar and best avoided.

Q) Should I have natural yoghurt with a fat meal or a carb meal?

A) If you have a fat meal you can have any kind of natural yoghurt – even full fat Greek yoghurt if you like it (or crème fraiche or fromage frais). With a carb meal you would need to have (very) low fat natural yoghurt /crème fraiche/fromage frais. This is why you can have skimmed milk with cereal, as the milk is so low fat it is OK to have with the carb. Not mixing fats and carbs takes a bit of effort, but it is so worth it, as this 'rule' really impacts weight loss.

If you want something with yoghurt for dessert, the one fruit that you can have after meals is berries – strawberries, raspberries, blackberries etc. Berries are so low in carbohydrate that they can be eaten with fat meals and they also don't cause bloating after eating other foods.

Q) What is hummus? What is that classed as?

A) Hummus is the Arabic word for chickpea, so this is the main ingredient in Hummus. Chickpeas are carbs, but Hummus is often made in a base of (olive) oil, so it also has a measurable fat content. In 100g of Hummus there are 20g of carbohydrate and 9g of fat.

Think of Hummus as a carb meal, therefore, but don't have 'lashings' of it with lots of brown bread, for example, or the fat content will start to add up. A good carb meal would be wholemeal pita bread stuffed with grated carrot, salad leaves, pepper slices and Hummus.

Hummus is full of protein, fibre and nutrients, so it is a healthy food. In 100g of Hummus, there are 4g of fibre and 5g of protein – so this is a good source of protein for Vegetarians.

Q) What about sweet potatoes? Are they the same as normal potatoes?

A) Yes. They should be treated as a staple carb, not as a 'free vegetable'. Sweet potatoes are actually higher in carbohydrate than normal potatoes (that shouldn't be a surprise – the word 'sweet' is a big clue). Sweet potatoes are 95% carb (5% protein) and normal potatoes are 92% carb. They are not allowed in Phase 1, therefore. In Phase 2, they should form the basis of a carb meal and be eaten with other carbs e.g. veggie chilli or with very low fat products, like virtually fat free cottage cheese.

I do get questions like – what about parsnips and other root vegetables? Are they not the same as potatoes? The key points here are:

- Carrots, for example, contain 10g of carb per 100g and sweet potatoes have got 20g of carb per 100g. So, potatoes are in a different carb league amongst the root vegetables. (Please note that water content makes the numbers look odd. When we say sweet potatoes are 95% carb, we mean, of the bit that is not water, 95% is carb i.e. there are 20g of carb and barely 1g of protein and the rest is water).

- Parsnips do have almost as high carb content as potatoes, but the quantities in which they are normally consumed are quite different. Whereas a baked potato can be 200g in weight, you are unlikely to serve yourself 200g of parsnips. If you were planning to have this quantity of parsnips, make sure you're having a carb meal.

Q) Are nuts and seeds allowed?

A) Nuts, seeds (and whole milk) are rare foods that have fat and carbohydrate in reasonable quantities. Most foods are carb/proteins or fat/proteins. (Isn't it interesting that nature naturally separates foods in this way?)

Nuts are natural foods (especially in shells), but I advise not eating them in Phase 1 or 2 because of the fat and carb content. Peanuts, as an example, have 51g of fat and 25g of carb in a 100g portion. Nuts can be eaten in Phase 3 with the usual 'not too much' and 'not too often' advice for cheating well.

I do advise people to think of food on a spectrum, rather than being black and white. On the spectrum of 'sugar is about as bad as you can get' and 'Salade Niçoise is about as good as you can get', nuts are definitely on the good side of the line, but they are best avoided while you are trying to lose weight. If you want to cheat, however, nuts are much better than all sweets and most crisps.

Seeds vary in composition, but are quite similar to nuts. The most common seeds, sunflower seeds, are predominantly fats. 100g of sunflower seeds has 51g of fat and 20g of carbohydrate. Seeds are also best avoided in quantities, therefore, until Phase 3.

A few nuts or seeds in (ideally) fat meal recipes will be fine. Just don't eat them by the bag-full as snacks, as one of my clients did, otherwise both the carb and fat intake will soon add up.

Q) What is Tofu made of?

A) Tofu comes from the soybean, just as cheese comes from milk. In 100g of Tofu there are 4g of fat and less than 1g of carbohydrate. So it is more fat than carb, but it is barely either. So Tofu can be eaten with cheese as a fat meal or with vegetables and beans as a carb meal.

We don't normally talk about protein, as we are more interested in fats and carbs. However, Tofu is an excellent source of Vegetarian protein. In 100g of Tofu there are 8g of protein. It is a great source of calcium and has all eight essential amino acids. The rest of the 100g, not accounted for, is water.

Q) What is Quorn made of? (Also known as Mycoprotein)

A) "*Myco*" is the Greek word for "*Fungi*", so Mycoprotein is effectively a fungus based protein. Immediately we can say that this is not good for anyone suffering from Candida. Quorn^{TM} is just the brand name for Mycoprotein.

Mycoprotein is made in fermenters similar to those used in a brewery. It is made by adding oxygen, nitrogen, glucose and minerals to a fungus called Fusarium venenatum.

I only recently discovered that glucose (sugar) was added in the process of making Mycoprotein. However, in 100g of Quorn, there are 3.5g of fat and 2g of carbohydrate, so there can barely be a trace of sugar in any serving (the sugar can only be a part of even the small part that is carbohydrate). As with Tofu, Quorn is more of a fat than a carb, but it is barely either. So it can be eaten as part of a fat or a carb meal.

In 100g of Quorn, there are 12g of protein, so it is a high protein alternative to meat for Vegetarians. It does have egg for binding, so it is not suitable for a Vegan. There are also nearly 5g of fibre in 100g of Quorn, so it is quite a good source of dietary fibre. In case you are wondering what makes up the rest, 75g out of 100g is water.

Overall, Quorn fails the basic 'food in the form that nature intends us to eat it' test, as it has been through a manufactured process. However, it can be a useful food to include in your diet if you don't suffer from Candida and particularly if you are Vegetarian and need extra food options.

2) The Harcombe Diet vs. traditional diet advice

Q) How is it different to other diets?

A) 1) It works! I set out to understand why we had an obesity epidemic and to design a diet that would eliminate hunger and food cravings. I did not set out to design a diet that would lose people 17lbs in five days and yet, at the time of going to print, this is the record for Phase 1. As a bonus, the most common themes in the endless testimonials are: *"I'm not hungry"*; *"My cravings have disappeared"*; *"I feel great"*; *"I've got more energy than I've ever known"* and *"This is the last diet I will ever need"*.

2) It fundamentally rejects the calorie theory, upon which 99% of diets are based. The other 1% of diets are the very low carb Atkins and Co. These will work, if you can stick to them. If you don't want the bad breath, constipation and boredom that tend to go with them, you may like this diet.

The 99% will not work, and we have a century's worth of obesity journals to prove this. (Sales of all diet books would have ceased decades ago if calorie counting did work). One definition of madness is to do the same thing again and again and to expect a different result. To go on a calorie restricted diet, is therefore, mad.

The Harcombe Diet is so simple; for centuries it was accepted as the only way to eat. It is based on the principle that nature knows best. Not government or public health agencies, not food manufacturers – nature.

On this diet, we eat only real food – food in the form that nature intends us to eat it. We eat this natural food in sufficient quantities to nourish our body and at regular intervals to give the body no reason to store fat. We don't eat processed food – food in the form that food manufacturers intend us to eat it.

3) The new and unique contribution of The Harcombe Diet is the discovery that there are three very common medical conditions that cause insatiable food cravings and that these conditions, in turn, are caused by eating less (i.e. calorie restricted diets).

The Harcombe Diet has been carefully designed to be the perfect diet to overcome all three conditions. These conditions, by the way, come with a whole range of other, nasty, symptoms. So, if you just want to lose weight, this book will tell you how. If you want to get rid of things as wide ranging as dandruff or waking up at 4am – this book could help you with way more than your waistline.

I've been asked by the media – if you don't agree with the "*Eat less, do more*" advice – what do you agree with? My answer is "*Eat better and do whatever you like*".

I've also been asked – is the diet low carb or low fat and the answer is neither. It is real food – carbs and fats – in whatever quantities you want – just not at the same meal. But you know that by now.

Q) Why haven't I been able to stick to a diet?

A) Because you have had cravings that are so strong you might as well have been a drug addict trying to give up heroin or a smoker trying to give up cigarettes. You are not weak-willed or greedy. You are fighting a force on an hourly basis that would beat the strongest of wills.

You have these cravings because of one thing that you have been doing and because of one, or all, of three conditions that you may have:

- The one thing that you have been doing is calorie counting/trying to eat less. As soon as you try to eat less fuel than your body needs, you will crave food, as this is your body's way of making you eat to give it the fuel that it needs.

- The conditions that you may have, which are causing your cravings, are Candida, Food Intolerance and Hypoglycaemia. Candida makes you crave sugary, yeasty and vinegary foods. Food Intolerance causes cravings for anything to which you are intolerant – this can literally be any food or drink from eggs to alcohol. Hypoglycaemia drives you to crave carbohydrates, especially processed carbs, as your blood glucose level rises and falls on an hourly basis. You need to eliminate processed carbohydrates and any foods to which you are intolerant, to overcome the cravings. Once the cravings subside you will then have the chance to reach a healthy weight and stay there long term.

Q) Why does everyone tell me to count calories?

A) Why do people smoke when it is a well-known fact that smoking kills one in two people who use the product, over time, exactly as it is intended to be used by the manufacturers? I struggle to answer this one as it just doesn't make sense. I think just as it has taken us years to realise that smoking is probably the worst thing we can do for our health, so it will take us years to get rid of the calorie myth.

Governments, doctors and dieticians have become so comfortable with the little slogan "*Eat less, do more*", they seem to have become blind to the fact that, not only is it not working, we are actually becoming fatter by the year.

People tell you to count calories because they think that if your body takes in less fuel than it needs you will lose weight. You now know that if you take in less fuel than your body needs the first thing that your body will do is to crave food to get you to eat more. The next thing that your body will do is to become weaker, less healthy and less able to resist problems such as Candida, Food Intolerance and Hypoglycaemia and then your cravings will get even worse. You also know that if you count calories you will simply slow down your metabolism, making weight loss harder still.

One of the most important things to take out of this book is a changed way of thinking. If you read this book and still think counting calories is the answer I have failed and you will continue to fail. You **must** throw out this myth and see how counting calories leads to food cravings, lower metabolism and increased weight rather than reduced weight.

Q) Why can't I still count calories?

A) Because if you continue to count calories you will continue to try to restrict them. If you start to find yourself eating 2000 calories a day, or more, you will consciously, or subconsciously, try to cut back. The hardest thing that you will do, in following the eating advice in this book, is to give up your 'prop' of counting calories.

Your key goal now is to stop cravings, not to count calories. If you try to eat fewer calories than your body needs you will crave food and it is the food cravings that are making you overweight. After reading this book, if you still think calories make you fat then eat no carbohydrate whatsoever for a few days. Eat as much fat/protein as you like and see how much weight you lose. I expect it will be pounds. Then ask yourself how you can eat so many calories and still lose weight – because calories are fuel for your body not bad things that make you fat.

Q) Won't I put on weight if I don't count calories?

A) No. You will put on weight if you continue to crave food like an addict and give into those cravings. Your number one objective now has to be to stop cravings, not to count calories. Put all your effort into stopping cravings by getting your Candida, Food Intolerance and Hypoglycaemia under control and don't waste any effort on counting calories. You are going to stop eating the foods that have been making you fat, so you will not put on weight. You will be nourishing your body and giving it what it needs, which is going to help it find its natural and healthy weight.

Also, don't forget that on this diet you don't eat empty calories – no sugar, trans fats or refined carbohydrates. So, all of your calories are going to 'count' – they are going to nourish you and give you vitamins and minerals, not just calories. This will make a huge difference to your health and weight.

Q) Should I count carbohydrates...?

A) No! Don't count anything – just put all that energy that used to be spent counting calories into craving control. Your number one goal now is to stop cravings. Do that and everything else will follow.

Q) I have been told if I stop eating certain things I will crave them more – many diets advise me to have a little bit of what I fancy – why is this book saying to avoid certain foods?

A) How crazy is this? Is the heroin addict told to have just a bit of heroin but not too much? Is the alcoholic told to have just one drink but not the whole bottle? The food addict would be a lot better off if they could go cold turkey on food, just as the drug addict, alcoholic and smoker can go cold turkey on their addiction. We can't stop eating, but we can stop eating certain foods – the ones causing us problems. Sugar does nothing positive for our health whatsoever, so we will lose nothing by giving it up. Similarly there are wholemeal alternatives for all processed carbohydrates and we will always be better off nutritionally by eating the wholemeal alternatives to processed foods.

Having read this book you should know that you are craving food because of one, or all, of calorie counting, Candida, Food Intolerance or Hypoglycaemia. Your cravings will get steadily worse, unless you stop eating the foods that are causing these conditions and food cravings. Remember that the 'devil' in your head is telling you to eat the food(s) to which you are addicted so this voice will jump on any magazine article that says that you can eat a bit of what you fancy. This is what you want to believe.

The time to have "*a little bit of what you fancy*" is when you are at your natural weight and when you are free from Candida, Food Intolerance and Hypoglycaemia and your immune system is able to cope with processed carbohydrates. Until then, a little bit of what you fancy will lead to a lot of what you fancy and it will keep you where you are now.

Q) I have also been told to 'graze' – to eat little and often. Why is that and should I do it?

A) There has been a lot of diet advice in recent years that you should eat little and often. I still can't believe how often I see this advice in the media. "*Keep your blood sugar level topped up throughout the day*", is advised. Assuming that people would eat carbohydrates, little and often, and not pure fat and protein, all this will achieve is that the pancreas will be overworked trying to keep your blood glucose level in the normal range. Your blood glucose level should be kept stable and normal to keep your body happy – any 'topping up' just has to be corrected with a dose of insulin.

Now that you know that insulin is the fattening hormone you know that the fewer times you raise your blood glucose level during the day, the better. If you graze, especially if you graze on low fat foods, which are generally high carbohydrate foods, then you are causing your body to release insulin on a more regular basis and this is what will make you fat.

Q) Remind me why this insulin thing is so important?

A) The key thing to take away from this book is that it is insulin, not calories, which makes you fat. Insulin is a hormone that is released by the pancreas (an organ in your body) when you eat something that raises your blood glucose level. Only carbohydrates raise your blood glucose level. Fats have no impact on your blood glucose level at all and therefore the body does not release any insulin when you eat fat on its own. The pancreas releases insulin to get your blood glucose level back to 'normal'. If it didn't do this you would be diabetic.

When we eat carbohydrates, our body decides how much of the energy taken in is needed immediately and how much should be stored for future requirements. As our blood glucose level rises, insulin is released from the pancreas and this insulin converts some of the glucose to glycogen. Glycogen is our energy store room. If all the glycogen storage areas are full, insulin will convert the excess to fatty tissue. This is why insulin has been called the fattening hormone.

Q) How do I start this diet?

A) Start Phase 1 as soon as you a) have read this book, b) know why you crave food, c) are prepared to stop counting calories and d) are prepared to start a journey that will change your life. Don't come up with excuses for not starting it. Every day that you delay, your cravings will get worse and the battle will be that much harder when you do start it.

Q) When do I move on to different phases?

A) You can stay on Phase 1 as long as you like and this is recommended for people showing strong signs of all of the conditions. Phase 1 can be followed safely and healthily indefinitely. Phase 2 widens your food choices and can make the eating plan more enjoyable and flexible. When you move on to Phase 2 really take care not to re-introduce foods that you have been craving.

Q) Can I go back to Phase 1?

A) Yes. You can dip back into Phase 1 and do another five day burst whenever you feel like it (as a detox, or as an extra weight loss boost). This is a great idea if you hit a plateau and want a fresh kick start.

Q) Weight loss – Is it the same as other diets, i.e. 1-2 lbs a week or can I expect less/more?

A) I think you'll find that you don't lose 1-2lbs a week on other diets, or you wouldn't have a weight problem! Phase 1 weight loss has been consistently high and spectacular in some cases. Phase 2 really does vary for every individual – there is no formula in the world when it comes to weight loss. I really wish that there were, but there just isn't. Some people have lost 3-5 pounds a week in Phase 2, some have lost a few pounds one week then plateaued for a while and then lost more. The key thing is, that you will lose weight steadily and keep it off. Even when people start cheating (a little bit) they rarely put the weight back on, so I have lots of case studies who seem happy to lose weight, then plateau/cheat, then lose a bit more. Some are dipping back into Phase 1 for a re-boost after a few weeks. I love it when people play with the diet and make it their own.

Q) How will I feel on The Harcombe Diet?

A) In Phase 1 you might feel quite unwell – like having a mild flu. You may have headaches from food addiction withdrawal. You may feel lethargic and you may have little interest in the foods that are allowed, as what you really want are the other foods – the ones that you crave. You are likely to have unbelievable cravings, but just take each day at a time, each hour at a time if necessary, and the cravings absolutely will subside.

By the end of Phase 1 (for some people after just two to three days) you could start feeling fantastic – more mentally alert and clear headed than you have done for ages. You should notice your skin has a lovely natural colour, not the red, blotchy colour you get when you keep eating foods to which you are intolerant. Your eyes will sparkle and you should sleep better than you have done for ages (not a carbohydrate induced stupor from which you wake feeling sluggish).

In Phase 2 you should feel great. The cravings will be barely noticeable. You may still **want** your previous favourites, but you won't have an overwhelming craving for them as you have had in the past. You really will be able to take them or leave them. Don't be fooled too early into thinking you can eat them again and not have the cravings return. You need to get to your natural weight, and realise how wonderful life is when you are slim and energetic and free from food addiction, before you can make an informed choice about whether or not to have the 'forbidden' foods again.

In Phase 3 you should feel free. The key thing about Phase 3 is that you have the freedom to eat what you want **almost** when you want and you will have the tools to stay in control. You will find that you get to the point where you are making sober and informed choices. When you are genuinely **not** craving processed carbohydrates you will find it easy to reject them in favour of foods that fill you up and make you feel good. For the first time in your life, you will control your eating; your eating won't control you.

Q) How much effort will this be?

A) How does the well-known saying go? – *you don't get something for nothing*. If you really want to be slim, more than you want to eat, you now have the knowledge and tools to achieve this. You know you just have to stop the cravings and then your eating can be back in your control. Phase 1 will be an effort, but it is just five days long. No time at all, in terms of the rest of your life. Put all your remaining willpower into those five days and your cravings will be manageable by the end of Phase 1.

Phase 2 should be not much effort at all. It will almost seem unfair that you are not hungry, that you are eating healthy foods, feeling full of life and energy and still losing weight.

Phase 3 is as much or as little effort as you make it. If you don't cheat too much, or too often, you will find your cravings easy to manage and you will love the freedom of being able to cheat and have others wonder how you stay so slim.

What you will find is that if you cheat too much, or too often, the cravings will return and then you will have to go back to where you are now to fight the food addiction and cravings that return. You will then need to return to Phase 1 or Phase 2 to get back in control.

Q) What will be the benefits?

A) Almost too many to list:

- Feeling good about nourishing and nurturing your body, rather than stuffing and starving it;

- Feeling high energy and a real zest for life;

- Reaching and maintaining a healthy weight;

- Having sparkling eyes, clear skin, sleeping well and feeling good;

- Having a strengthened immune system enabling you to resist infections, colds and flu that others are susceptible to;

- Feeling you control food rather than that food controls you;

- No longer feeling afraid of food, no longer avoiding social events because you are concerned about food or your weight.

Q) What if I don't do something?

A) Sadly food addiction is not a steady state that you can decide to tackle in weeks, months or years time. Every day that you continue to feed Candida, eat foods to which you are intolerant, or upset your blood glucose level, you are making your food addiction, cravings and health worse. The longer you leave it before tackling your food addiction the worse it will get. I cannot urge you strongly enough – **tackle it now** – before it gets any worse and, therefore, even harder to tackle. Do something and the rest of your life starts now.

Q) What do I do if I eat something that is not good for me?

A) Don't start a binge. Get back on track. Don't let one small slip ruin all the efforts you have made. To minimise the damage done, drink lots of water to enable your body to flush through more easily. If the thing that you have eaten is something that will cause a sharp rise (and fall) in blood glucose level then watch out for the fall and don't let this lead to further cravings. Just as you feel your blood glucose high is wearing off, eat a piece of fruit or a wholemeal carbohydrate (e.g. a sugar-free oat biscuit) to help your blood glucose level rise gently when it is about to crash down.

If what you have eaten triggers cravings, you may need to return to Phase 1 until the cravings subside again.

Finally, try to learn from what has happened. Why did you eat something that wasn't good for you? Have the cravings returned? If so why? Is Candida still a problem for you? Are you in the first few days of Phase 1 and the cravings are unbearable? If so, re-read Chapter 12 and see how you can get through the five days next time. Unless you plan to exist, not live, you will have to tackle this some time so do it now. Are you in Phase 3 and have you been cheating too much and/or too often? If so, return to Phase 2 until you feel in control again and cut back on your cheating next time. It really is trial and error until you know what you can get away with.

Q) How healthy is The Harcombe Diet?

A) The Harcombe Diet tells you not to eat processed foods. These are foods with a lot of the nutrients and goodness removed, so we are actually much better off and much healthier for not eating these. This diet lets you eat all natural foods that are full of nutrients like meat, fish, dairy products, vegetables, salad, fruit and whole grains. Finally, this diet doesn't make you hungry, or send your body into starvation mode. I cannot think of a healthier diet.

Q) Please do you have more recipes available?

A) All the recipes needed for the Phase 1 and Phase 2 *"Planner"* menus, are in this book.

The Harcombe Diet Recipe Book accompanies *The Harcombe Diet Book*. This has been co-written with Rachel McGuinness, chef and founder of *"The Life Spa"*. There are over 250 recipes in this book – all categorised into carb vs. fat meals and those suitable for Candida, Food Intolerance, Hypoglycaemia and/or Vegetarians.

I also recommend *Cooking Without* and *Cooking Without for Vegetarians* by Barbara Cousins. These really are excellent books for anyone looking to eat real food without wheat/dairy/sugar, or to have these foods highlighted where they are used.

3) Candida, Food Intolerance & Hypoglycaemia

Q) Why is fruit restricted in the diets for Candida?

A) The advice on Candida to date has been to restrict fruit totally for a few weeks and quite significantly for some time thereafter. This advice is given because fruit is a carbohydrate and any carbohydrate, especially sweet fruits, can feed the yeast. Starving the yeast of the foods it needs to survive means avoiding all sugars, including fruit sugar, for a period of time.

The advice varies in terms of the period for which fruit sugar should be avoided. Some practitioners advise weeks, if not months, without fruit. This undoubtedly will help with Candida, but there are more factors to consider in relation to your overall wellbeing. In this book we avoid fruit just for Phase 1, to have a quick and significant impact on Candida. We then advise no more than 1-2 pieces of fruit a day, in Phase 2, for as long as Candida is a problem for you.

If you are not that keen on fruit, then you can continue to avoid it for as long as Candida causes you a problem. However, if you like fruit, it is more important for your diet to be enjoyable, practical and something you can stick to. Many people, women in particular, would simply not start a diet that advised them to avoid fruit for weeks.

Health is an all over concept and if someone is happy and enjoying their food, this is almost as valuable as forcing someone to eat 'the perfect diet', whatever that may be. You need to become your own health monitor and balance enjoyment of healthy foods with the knowledge and awareness of foods that cause you problems. If fruit does you more harm than good then restrict it, if not, enjoy it.

Q) How long should the 'die-off' last (with Candida?)

A) This very much depends on how severe your Candida problem has become. If you have read this book in good time and are tackling the problem early, you may find the first five days uncomfortable but not bad enough to make you feel very unwell. If you have been overeating and craving food for years and have always wondered why, and you now realise that Candida is one of your problems, you could be in for quite a rough time. You could experience die-off for many days or even a few weeks, so be prepared to launch a war on this unwelcome invader.

Try to view 'die-off' as a positive thing – the worse you feel, the more harm you are doing to the yeast and the more you are killing it off. Use the pain of the 'die-off' to strengthen your resolve to rid your body of this parasite and to never let it return. See 'die-off' as proof that Candida has been a problem for you and look forward to the time when the yeast and cravings will be back under control and your overeating and excess weight will disappear.

Q) Will I have Candida for ever?

A) Yes and No. You will always have Candida in your body, as it lives within all of us. However, you can get this parasite back in control and stop the huge impact it is having on your health and wellbeing. The best way to keep Candida at bay is to keep your immune system strong and healthy by eating well, taking a vitamin and mineral tablet daily, doing some exercise regularly that you enjoy and getting balance in your work and play.

Q) Is there a medical test for Candida?

A) Some nutritionists do offer stool tests, which can detect levels of Candida in the matter excreted by the body. Unless you have a huge desire to send away a 'number two' in a medical container I would advise sticking to the questionnaire in Chapter 3, as this will give you a very good idea of whether or not Candida is an issue for you.

There are some Candida support organisations that offer information on blood and saliva tests that are available. You can find one on the Internet.

I have also heard of a Do-It-Yourself test for Candida. The test involves spitting into a clear glass of water first thing in the morning and seeing what happens within the next half an hour. If there are 'strings' coming down from your saliva, or if the water turns cloudy, or if your saliva sinks to the bottom of the glass, this has been shown to be a good indication that you have an overgrowth of Candida.

Q) When can I re-introduce more foods?

A) As soon as you know that Candida is not a problem for you (redo the questionnaire in Chapter 3 and see if the many symptoms have subsided), you can re-introduce more foods cautiously to make sure that you keep the Candida under control. Try introducing foods one at a time so that, if the symptoms do return, you will know what has caused this to happen. If they don't return, this is an excellent sign that your immune system is doing well, having been nourished with healthy food.

Q) Is there any medication for Candida?

A) Pessaries for thrush in women have been available for some time. Oral medication for Candida used to be available on prescription only, but there are now over-the-counter tablet remedies available at pharmacies. These are not to be taken regularly, but they offer 'one tablet' options for Candida, which work throughout the whole body and digestive tract. The Pharmacist can advise you.

Q) Why do Food Intolerances vary from country to country?

A) The key cause of Food Intolerance is eating too much of any one substance too often. Hence the foods most often consumed in each country and in the largest quantities are the ones most likely to cause Food Intolerance. In Australia the foods eaten most of and most often are wheat and milk – the same as in the UK. In the US they are dairy foods, wheat, corn, eggs, soy, peanuts and sugar. In Taiwan they are rice and soya beans.

Q) What if I have none of the conditions, or only one or two of them?

A) The fewer conditions you have the better for you. You may have read this book in time and caught things before they get too bad. You may have none of the conditions and are craving food just because you have been calorie counting and, therefore, need more petrol in your tank (you are just hungry). If you only have Candida then you will need to avoid yeast, sugar and vinegar in Phase 2 but you may find you are able to tolerate wheat for example. If you only have a particular Food Intolerance, such as milk, then avoid that food in Phase 2. If you don't crave any particular foods (which would suggest Food Intolerance) and you don't think Candida is a problem for you but you are getting strong swings in your blood glucose level then it may be just Hypoglycaemia that you need to think about. The fewer conditions you have, the more options for food you have in Phase 2.

4) Cravings

Q) How does Candida cause food cravings?

A) Candida is a living organism and every living thing has a natural self-preservation mechanism – we all fight to survive. The yeast living inside us is no exception. When Candida really takes hold you will crave the foods that feed the yeast to ensure it grows and flourishes – all processed carbohydrates, sugary foods, concentrated fruit sugar, yeast and yeast derivatives and vinegary/pickled foods. There is evidence to suggest that yeast itself does not feed the yeast but the consumption of bread and other foods containing yeast generally maintains the environment that the yeast needs to thrive in your body.

Q) How does Food Intolerance cause food cravings?

A) The real irony is that the foods to which you are intolerant are the foods that you crave. Just as the drug addict or smoker craves their fix so you crave the substance that is causing you harm. It starts off with a particular food or drink that you consume on regular occasions. Any substance that you eat daily can start to cause problems and those you eat several times a day are the chief suspects. It takes three to four days for a substance to pass through our bodies, so we can overload our bodies if we eat a substance daily or even more often.

Our bodies then literally become 'intolerant' to the food – i.e. they can't cope with any more of it. You would think that we would shun the food if we had become intolerant to it but in fact the addiction that goes with Food Intolerance actually means that the opposite happens. If we remember back to the definition of addiction we go through these characteristics with Food Intolerance:

- We start with an uncontrollable craving;

- We then need more and more of the offending substance in order to get the same 'high' i.e. more cravings;

- We develop physical and/or psychological dependence, more cravings still;

- We suffer from the adverse effects.

Q) How does Hypoglycaemia cause food cravings?

A) This is a really simple one. As soon as your blood glucose level falls below normal, your body will cry out for food. It will crave any food but, most likely, sweet foods to get your blood glucose level back up again. When your hands are shaking, you feel a bit sweaty, a bit light headed or even faint in extreme cases, this is your body begging you to eat. You reach for a confectionery bar and immediately feel better, almost euphoric, as your blood glucose level shoots up. However, the confectionery bar is alien to your pancreas, so your body produces too much insulin, your blood glucose level falls below normal again and the cravings continue.

Q) Why do I have to stop eating the foods I most like?

A) Because these are the foods you most crave and you crave foods that are causing you problems – this is the real irony of Candida, Food Intolerance and Hypoglycaemia. The foods you don't crave are not causing you problems. This is why meat, fish, eggs, vegetables, brown rice and Natural Live Yoghurt are generally OK for anyone – they are hardly ever the subject of cravings.

Q) Why have I had these cravings?

A) If you have been calorie counting you have probably just been hungry. Because of your body's incredible survival instinct, it has been trying to get you to eat (anything) just to maintain the fuel levels that it needs to survive. The activity of calorie counting alone has led to cravings.

On top of this, calorie counting has depleted your nutrients and weakened your immune system. This, with or without other factors such as taking the birth control pill, or antibiotics or having had extreme stress, can lead to any, or all, of Candida, Food Intolerance and Hypoglycaemia. You only need one of these conditions and you will have cravings as strong as any faced by a drug addict.

Q) Will cravings go away?

A) Yes. This is within your control. First you need to stop calorie counting. This may require a change in your mind set, but you have nothing to lose and everything to gain. Then all of the conditions – Candida, Food Intolerance and Hypoglycaemia – can be controlled in the short and long term. The other thing to remember is, if you don't start to control these conditions they will only get worse. So the sooner you tackle this, the better. Look at the tips for positive thinking in Chapter 12 and be determined to crack this. One of the best tips for motivation is that, unless you plan to live your entire life overweight and exhausted, you are going to have to crack this some time. Why not start now?

Q) When will they go away?

A) The good news is that you can significantly reduce food cravings quite quickly. In just five days you can do the following:

- You can stop counting calories and thereby stop your body demanding fuel;

- You can have a major impact on the Candida overgrowth in your body and dramatically reduce the cravings for yeasty, vinegary and sugary foods;

- You can eliminate the foods to which you are intolerant and clear any traces of these from your system, leading to a dramatic reduction in cravings;

- You can stabilise your blood glucose level in fewer than five days – even a day's healthy eating can start the stabilisation of your blood glucose level.

The first five days will be tough, but you really can achieve a dramatic reduction in cravings in this short time period. Without the cravings trying to ruin your good intentions, your willpower is free to take you to the success you have always dreamed of.

Q) How do I stop 'good' days and 'bad' days?

A) By this you mean bingeing and starving. The key is to stop either one of 'good' days or 'bad' days as one leads directly to the other. You only try to have a 'good' day to lose the weight you gain after a 'bad' day. And you only have bad days when you are so hungry and deprived after a 'good day' of calorie restriction. It doesn't matter which one you vow to stop – starve days or binge days – one leads to the other so stopping one stops the other.

Q) How do I stop being a food addict?

A) By stopping the food cravings. This in turn is done by stopping calorie counting and by making sure that any problems you have with Candida, Food Intolerance and/or Hypoglycaemia are addressed. You must stop eating the foods that you crave – easier said than done I hear you say and you are right – but this is the only way to stop the food cravings. Now that you understand what you crave and why, you have the power to overcome food addiction.

Q) I have hit a problem with cheese, I can't stop eating it. My craving for chocolate is long gone, but has now been replaced by cheese. What do you suggest I do? Thanks in advance.

A) The way to get rid of any craving is to **not** eat the substance for at least five days. Remember how tough those five days are but your craving really does go as soon as the substance has passed through the body.

Cheese is an interesting craving because it is a fat/protein so this is quite rare. Cheese has no effect on Hypoglycaemia, so this is not the problem. Cheese can feed Candida, but I suspect that the problem that has returned is Food Intolerance. You may need to come off all dairy products for a while, so that you are not feeding the craving for cheese in another way (via milk or yoghurt for example). Natural Live Yoghurt should still be OK, because of the many health benefits that this has, but have a goat's or sheep's version of NLY just to be safe.

Q) I am puzzled why I have sugar cravings straight after eating a meal. I just ate a carbohydrate meal consisting of brown rice and spinach, so I should not feel anything. Is this normal? Or is this connected to Candida, Food Intolerance and low blood sugar?

A) First of all, brown rice and spinach are nutritious foods so well done for choosing them.

There is unlikely to be any Food Intolerance, as neither of these foods are common intolerances.

You could have a bad case of Candida, in which case even brown rice can feed the Candida to a slight extent (just because it is a carb). This is also unlikely though, unless you have eaten a mountain of brown rice. It may not be the rice feeding the Candida, but just that Candida is still rampant in your body and it is generally craving sweet things.

My chief suspect would be Hypoglycaemia. If your blood glucose handling mechanism is not working well, your body could over-react to any carbohydrates eaten. In this case, your blood glucose level could rise, after eating rice, and then not be controlled appropriately with your pancreas releasing insulin. If your blood glucose handling mechanism is overly sensitive, any carbs can upset your blood glucose balance and this can lead to sugar cravings.

I would recommended sticking with the plan, as your body can only get better avoiding processed foods and eating whole grains and healthy, natural foods. Your immune system will get stronger, so stick with it and be determined to conquer those three conditions.

I would stay off very sweet fruits for a few weeks and then start slowly on a small banana or a few grapes to test if you can tolerate 'higher sugar' fruits. Stick to 1-2 pieces of fruit a day in the early stage of Phase 2 and stick to apples, pears, oranges and lower sugar fruits.

I would also recommend that you take a good multi vitamin/mineral tablet and you may like to take a chromium supplement of 200µg daily, as this is the mineral that really helps with blood glucose balance and sugar cravings.

Q) This is my 7th day on Phase 1, and I do feel great, and for the first time in ages, I'm able to sleep at night. However, I can't believe how much I am craving chocolate. The reason I am still on Phase 1 is because I am afraid to leave it, because my cravings for chocolate are still so strong. I feel lost without chocolate, but am hoping that eventually the cravings will subside. My questions are:

- Is it normal to still be obsessed with chocolate after the 5 days?

- Will choosing to stick to Phase 1 help banish cravings more so than if I moved on to Phase 2?

Zoë I consider this the hardest, and most important thing I've done so far in life, and I cannot imagine a life that isn't obsessed with eating.

I tried Phase 1 a few times before and 'given in' around day 3 every time!

I've read all the positive testimonials, but my truth is that I'm finding this tearjerkingly hard!

So Zoë, should I continue with Phase 1?

A) Wow! Do you need any more proof that you are addicted to something you eat? You are doing SO well. I really can understand giving in on Phase 1 – the cravings are so strong that it is so hard not to. The thing is – you have to break the addiction sometime, otherwise it will always be there. I spent about 12 years addicted to food (age 16-28) and the years since not at all addicted and really enjoying food and there is just no comparison as to which is more enjoyable and liberating. You can get there too...

Stick with Phase 1 for as long as you can bear it. The strength of your cravings indicates all three conditions are highly likely, so you need to really get these under control. Candida is always the one that takes the longest time to overcome, so the longer you can attack this with Phase 1, the better.

When you feel the cravings are well under control, try a 'Phase 1 plus' and gradually re-introduce things that are allowed in Phase 2, but slowly and not eating too much of the re-introduced foods. e.g. don't go to unlimited fruit – maybe have one or two pieces a day. I would advise staying off wheat for a few weeks longer, as almost every person I have ever worked with has had a problem with wheat and this can cause cravings to return too quickly. Stick with rice pasta and rice based products for a while, but don't worry about limiting your rice quantity, as you did in strict Phase 1. (Don't forget in Phase 2 though, you are no longer allowed to mix fats and carbs, so a rice meal is a carb meal).

Other tips are:

- Has this coincided with the time of the month? Cravings for chocolate do increase during pre-menstrual time, because the body is craving iron and real chocolate is a good source of iron;

- You may like to take a good multi vitamin/mineral tablet daily, so that you are sure that you are getting the nutrients you need;

- Try increasing your intake of iron rich foods - spinach, red meat, dark green leaf vegetables, dried apricots – the latter in moderation, because they are processed fruits in effect.

The final tip may be a bit strange, but are you craving proper chocolate? If you are craving milk chocolate etc then it is more likely sugar or milk that you are craving (therefore avoid these products and your cravings will subside). A good way to test if you are craving cocoa is to get some 100% cocoa powder from the supermarket and see if that satisfies your craving – if it does – then it is pure cocoa you are addicted to. To give you hope – I used to have a clear intolerance to cocoa and my immune system has been strong enough for the last 10 years that it causes me no problems at all. I can have 85%+ cocoa chocolate every day and enjoy it without craving it.

You can get 99% cocoa chocolate from food halls and you can get 85% and 86% versions in supermarkets. If you think you can eat real chocolate, in moderation, without ruining your healthy diet, then build this into your Phase 2.

I have worked with lots of people who have a square or two of real chocolate after their two main meals of the day and they then have no desire to have a dessert or snack in between meals. Remember the signs of addiction though – if you get to the point that you need more than a couple of squares, if it is giving you a real physiological impact when you eat it, if you want it earlier and earlier each day – then your immune system is just not ready and you need to stay off it, get healthy and then you can return to it.

You really can be slim and eat quality chocolate – you've just got to go through a 'get healthy and stop being addicted' phase first.

Q) In two days time I'll be moving onto Phase 2, and I'm really looking forward to eating fruit again. I'm concerned with the 'no vegetable juices allowed' rule. I make my own juices and don't know if I'll be able to cope without my carrot, celery, cucumber and apple juice, or even my strawberry, blueberry, banana and orange juice, which I mix with live yoghurt for a fab breakfast. Do I have to ban them?

A) The first rule in Phase 2 is no processed foods and this is about not altering the food from its natural state. Although delicious and 'healthy', fruit and vegetable juices are processed in some way. When you have carrot juice, you are removing the juice of the carrot and leaving all the pulp (fibre) in the juicer. This will have an impact on your sugar handling system (pancreas etc) – not as bad as having a confectionery bar, but not as good as eating the whole raw carrot.

The strict answer is therefore – don't have them. The more flexible answer is, you could try the juices (vegetable first and then fruit if this is OK) and see if the cravings return. My worry is that they will, because you said you are really looking forward to eating fruit again. Fruit was one of the foods I most craved and found hardest to give up. The trouble is – Candida loves it, Hypoglycaemia comes from it and occasionally people are intolerant to fruit – oranges especially. To be safe I would stay off juices but, if you do try them, watch the cravings like a hawk and stop having the juices if the cravings return. Try having a slow release carb with the juice, if you do risk it, (e.g. porridge oats and veggie juice as a carb breakfast) and this may help with any sugar rush.

5) Specific foods (beyond the Top 10)

Q) Which **cereal** can I have for breakfast?

A) If wheat is not a problem for you, you can have shredded wheat, or bite size shredded wheat – 100% whole wheat. However, the vast majority of people I have worked with have had wheat as a Food Intolerance. So, it is best avoided for a few weeks in Phase 2 for most people. Thanks to gluten intolerance, there are many wheat-free alternatives to every-day foods in the supermarkets.

A great way to start the day is the way I do every morning – porridge. Get 100% oats – fine or jumbo, organic or normal – whatever you like. You can then add water or milk – again according to taste and whether or not you have milk Food Intolerance. Water makes this the fastest breakfast possible. In the time it takes to boil the kettle you can put some dry oats in a bowl and you then just pour the boiling water on top and stir in. For a quick version with milk, boil the milk in a pan or microwave, and then pour this on top of the oats. If you like your porridge mushy, you can then microwave the mixture for a minute or two to really let the liquid soak in. If you are sure that you are not suffering from Candida or Hypoglycaemia, you can add some chopped fresh fruit.

Rice cereal is another alternative. Health food shops have packets of 100% brown rice cereal, puffed into bits like sugar puffs, but without the sugar. It tastes great and is nice and crunchy for people who like crunchy food. A good brand is *Kallo*® and this is now in supermarkets as well as health food shops.

Remember, any cereal is a carb meal so you can only have it with skimmed milk. No whole milk is allowed, because that would be mixing your fats and carbs.

Q) I chew **sugar-free gum** and it says on the packet that it is high in carbs, but that the carbs are "sugars 0%" and "polyols 100%". What are polyols and where do they fit in with refined/unrefined carbs?

A) Polyols are carbohydrates and they are sugar-free sweeteners. Unlike highly concentrated sweeteners, like aspartame, which is used in very small amounts, polyols are used in the same quantity as sucrose (table sugar).

The most widely used polyols are sorbitol, mannitol and maltitol. (You will see these ingredients listed on various products). Sorbitol comes from glucose, mannitol from fructose, and maltitol from high maltose corn syrup.

Polyols come from sugars, but they are not processed by the body like sugars. The manufacturers claim that Polyols have advantages over sugar – fewer calories (we don't care about that); reduced insulin response (that's more important) and do not promote tooth decay. Polyols invariably have a health warning on the packet – excess consumption can have a laxative effect – anyone who has mindlessly munched through a packet of sugar-free mints will know about this!

The only benefit of chewing sugar-free gum that I can think of is that it neutralises the acid in the mouth after eating and therefore helps avoid tooth decay. I have heard an argument that it stops you eating, but it is actually the opposite – you are effectively eating all day long. It continues to feed a desire for a sweet taste and sweeteners are not healthy or natural as products. If you must chew gum then do it for the tooth protection reason after a meal (better still clean your teeth), but don't chew all day long and ideally don't chew at all.

Q) Is there any way I can have **chips**?

A) Yes. The Harcombe Diet way to do chips – for Phase 2 – is to chop up whole potatoes, with the skins on, and bake them in the oven on a tray brushed with olive oil or stir-fry them in a very small amount of olive oil. This is a carb meal, so only other carbs go with this. You can have home-made (sugar-free) tomato sauce, but no Ketchup. Avoid the vinegar, also, if you have Candida. Watch potatoes generally if you have Hypoglycaemia, as they are high on the glycaemic index.

Q) **Corn flour**: Can we use corn flour for thickening?

A) Corn flour is fine to use as a thickener. Corn flour is the starch extracted from maize (corn) that is soaked and ground to separate the germ and the bran. It contains no gluten, so it is not going to feed any wheat intolerance. It is strictly a carbohydrate, rather than a fat. However, it is OK with fat meals, as it is used in such small quantities it won't matter.

Q) Can I eat **cream** ?

A) In Phase 1, no, because we avoid dairy products (other than Natural Live Yoghurt) in Phase 1.

In Phase 2, yes, have cream as part of a fat meal. Cream is 92% fat, 3% protein and 5% carbohydrate. Hence 95% of it has no impact on insulin. It falls into the fat category, therefore, and so you can eat it with anything else fat in Phase 2.

Q) Can we eat/use **crème fraiche** or **Fromage Frais**?

A) In Phase 1, no, because we avoid dairy products in Phase 1. In Phase 2, yes, have them with fat meals. Check the ingredients carefully to ensure that you are eating just 100% crème fraiche or fromage frais – no sweeteners or additives or anything else 'processed'.

Q) Can we use **mascarpone cheese**?

A) In Phase 1, no, because we avoid dairy products in Phase 1. In Phase 2, yes. It is a fat, so have it with fat meals.

Q) Is it OK to take **painkillers**? I had a horrendous headache for two days (caffeine withdrawal?) and in the end gave in to paracetamol. Was that OK?

For your information, I'm following the diet not to lose weight (I'm your height and size), but to reduce sugar cravings. I also suspect I suffer from Candida. Any advice would be appreciated.

A) Headaches tablets are fine and needing them is a sure sign that there are withdrawal symptoms going on – could be caffeine, as you suggested, but sugar is another chief culprit. If you have been craving sugar then all three conditions could be going on – a sugar Food Intolerance, Candida driven sugar cravings and Hypoglycaemia induced blood glucose lows – hence why sugar is the biggest baddie of all processed foods. (Paracetamol is the best headache tablet to take, by the way, as it is the gentlest on the stomach – ibuprofen can harm the stomach lining, which can lead to leaky gut syndrome and cause further Candida and Food Intolerance).

Candida is sadly the toughest condition to zap. Your blood glucose level will be stabilised within Phase 1 and any Food Intolerances will have passed through your system by then but Candida is the one that can take a bit more time. I would stay off wheat for a few weeks after Phase 1 (have porridge or sugar-free rice cereals for breakfast and rice pasta instead of whole wheat pasta) as I have yet to work with a person who didn't have wheat intolerance. I would also recommend just 1-2 pieces of fruit per day for a few weeks to keep fruit sugar to a minimum. This will avoid the Candida being 're-fed'.

Q) **Pasta** vs. rice – which is better?

A) Rice, for Europeans and Americans, is rarely a food to which we are intolerant, as we don't eat it often enough to become intolerant to it. Pasta, however, is often a food to which we are intolerant, as it is from the wheat family, which we tend to eat at every meal – breakfast cereal, toast, sandwiches, bread, pizza, beer and so on. It is quite likely, therefore, that you will need to avoid wheat in Phase 2, if these are the foods that you crave.

You can try some whole wheat pasta as part of Phase 2, but if you find it causes your lethargy or cravings to return, you will know you have identified a problem food. Try rice pasta instead (you may not be able to taste the difference). Try to make rice, rather than pasta, your main carbohydrate during Phase 2. Brown rice is so delicious and versatile as a grain. You can make paella, Chinese vegetable dishes, Mexican chilli style dishes, vegetable curries and so on. Remember rice is a carbohydrate meal so you must eat this with vegetables and not fat. You can use some vegetable fat in cooking – e.g. stir-fry vegetables in olive oil – but no other fat.

Q) I just have a quick question. There are a few terms we don't see in America much – what are **pulses**, for example?

A) Pulses is a group term used to describe peas, beans and lentils. This group of foods is protein and carbohydrate, with hardly any fat. So, if you have any of these with a meal, it needs to be a carb meal. I lived in the US for a while and you don't come across pulses much at all so, unless you're Vegetarian, don't worry too much about them. (You could find a good health food shop at some point in your new way of eating and experiment with some of these goodies. Nutritionally pulses have a lot to offer).

244

Q) What about **potatoes** – good or bad?

A) Potatoes have had a mixed reaction in diet books. The book *Potatoes not Prozac*, by Kathleen DesMaisons, shows how the natural serotonin in potatoes makes us feel good. Michel Montignac points to the high glycaemic index of potatoes and advises us not to go near them. The advice in this book is that the whole potato is OK (i.e. a jacket potato in its skin), as it is not processed, but the processed versions of potatoes are not OK – oven chips, crisps etc.

Baked jacket potatoes are a useful food for office workers, as people often have a baked potato bar near work and can, therefore, get a practical hot meal for lunch. Also, a lot of offices have microwaves and you can bring in partially baked potatoes to heat up at lunchtime. Remember the potato is a carbohydrate meal, so don't mix it with fat – no butter, therefore, or cheese. You can have low fat cottage cheese, salad, ratatouille or vegetables – you get the idea.

Q) **Tinned tomatoes**: are these OK?

A) Yes they are – we use them all the time. Read the label carefully and go for the ones that have chopped tomatoes as big a % as possible of the ingredients and concentrated juice as small as possible (labels often actually give the %). Someone asked me about citric acid in tomatoes and this is fine – it is just a preservative. Any tin with tomatoes, juice, citric acid, herbs (optional) and nothing else is just fine. I haven't found anyone yet who craves tinned tomatoes.

Q) Can I have **smoked fish**?

A) Not in Phase 1, but you can in Phase 2 if you are sure that Candida is not a problem for you. Candida likes smoked foods (meat and fish), as well as pickled foods, so don't feed the nasty monster.

Q) What should I have for **snacks**?

A) Please note that the ideal way of eating is to have three big meals a day, which fully satisfy you, and not to snack during the day. However, if you really need snacks in the morning or afternoon, here's what you can have...

Phase 1 – any of the allowed foods at any time of the day e.g. hardboiled eggs, Natural Live Yoghurt, crudités, slices of unprocessed meat etc.

Phase 2 – any of the snacks listed above, or fruit, or pure oat biscuits. Take care not to have fat snacks close to a carb meal, or vice versa. Allow 3-4 hours between mixing fats and carbs

Phase 3 – ideally stick to good snacks, like those above. Add in 70% (or higher) cocoa chocolate and wholemeal, sugar-free, cereal bars. However, you can eat anything that you want provided you follow the cheating guidelines.

Q) Can I use **stock cubes**?

A) Yes – even in Phase 1, the occasional stock cube will be fine. Read all the ingredients carefully and try to get cubes without wheat or sugar. However, if you are struggling to find any, just pick the one that has the wheat and sugar furthest down the ingredients list – the quantity will be so tiny, when you make up the stock, as to be not really worth bothering about. Remember you can also use natural vegetable juices after cooking vegetables and add rice flour as a thickener. You can also make your own sauces using garlic, onion and tomato.

Q) Can I have **sweet corn**?

A) Nature delivers sweet corn on the cob, so, strictly speaking, you should eat corn on the cob so that you are eating the whole food – all the chewy bits that tinned sweet corn takes out. (You can't have butter on corn on the cob, as this mixes fat with carbs).

Tinned or frozen sweet corn is OK, but it does have a high glycaemic index so it impacts blood glucose more than green vegetables and salads etc. As a general rule, brighter coloured vegetables tend to be higher in carbohydrate (butternut squash, carrots, sweet corn) and therefore they are best to eat more sparingly than green vegetables and salad, which can be eaten in large quantities.

If you suspect that you have Candida, sweet corn is best avoided for a few weeks and it doesn't help Hypoglycaemia much either. In the US, corn is also a major Food Intolerance – because Americans eat a lot of popcorn and corn chips – so it is a food eaten too much of and too often.

Q) As a snack can I have **vegetable crisps**?

A) Vegetable crisps are best kept as a very occasional treat, rather than a regular snack. They are processed vegetables, as they are not the state in which we normally find vegetables (they are the vegetable equivalent of dried fruit). A better carb snack would be a piece of fruit or a couple of oat biscuits.

Food is on a spectrum (it is not black and white) and vegetable crisps are better than confectionery and regular crisps, but not as good as, say, an apple.

Q) Can I put balsamic or other **vinegar** on salads?

A) In Phase 1, no, vinegar and pickled foods feed yeast and we are trying to attack the Candida parasite.

In Phase 2, yes, but only if you are sure that Candida is not a problem for you. The best way to test this is to see if you are just as keen to eat the salad without vinegar on it. If the answer is no, then you are craving the vinegar, it's as simple as that. Try olive oil or lemon juice as a dressing instead.

Q) Why do I need **vitamins** if I'm eating good food?

A) Great question – the answer is that you don't *need* to take a supplement, but you may like to think of one as an insurance policy – better to be safe, just in case. Even real food requires nutritious soil and farming for optimal nutrition and there is much evidence that we over work farm land, such that the soil is not as nutritious as it has been historically. If you eat locally produced, organic vegetables and salads, free range meat and eggs and fresh fish, you are unlikely to need extra vitamins and minerals. If you don't have absolute confidence in the nutritional sources of your food, you may like to take a supplement.

6) Carbs, fats, protein and mixing – clearing up any confusion

Carbs

Q) Why are carbohydrates the baddies?

A) Just to make this clear – carbohydrates are not the baddies. Processed carbohydrates are the baddies. Fruit, wholemeal grains and vegetables are all carbohydrates, but they have not been processed in the way that cakes, biscuits and microwave meals have been. Processed carbohydrates are the baddies for the following reasons:

- They are low in nutrients;

- They are alien to our bodies and most importantly to our pancreas;

- They stimulate the production of insulin, which is the fattening hormone;

- They contribute to Candida, Food Intolerance and Hypoglycaemia and these in turn can lead to food cravings and weight gain;

- If we consume processed carbohydrates we will either be overeating other foods to get the nutrients that we need, or we will be deficient in some nutrients.

Q) Why is sugar the number one baddie?

A) Because it does nothing positive for our bodies and it does a lot that is negative instead. It is the only substance that we eat or drink that gives us virtually no nutrients whatsoever and it uses up our stock of vitamins and minerals in its digestion. It upsets blood glucose balance, makes our bodies produce insulin (the fattening hormone) and gives us nothing back in return. Sugar is 'empty calories' so we still need to eat more calories to get the nutrients that we need. It also tastes so sweet that it disturbs our taste buds for naturally sweet foods like fruit and vegetables. There are far more serious allegations about sugar and its impact on our health, from cancer to heart disease, which you will find easily doing some (Internet) research. Check the site ownership carefully – the official sounding "Sugar Bureau", for example, is run by the sugar companies.

Q) How do I know real food from processed?

A) Think of how nature delivers the product: oranges grow on trees, cartons of orange juice don't; baked potatoes come from the ground, chips don't; fish swims in the sea, fish fingers don't. Always think how nature delivers the food and that's the form in which you need to eat it.

Fats

Q) Why is fat OK to eat?

A) We need fat for all the cells in our bodies. Without the fat that our bodies need, we will suffer from all kinds of health complaints from minor ones, such as dry skin, to major ones such as strokes or stunted growth. Fat has got its bad reputation from the calorie myth (amongst other myths), in that people think if fat has nine calories per gram and carbohydrate has four calories per gram then we are better off eating carbohydrate. We now know that the calorie theory doesn't work, that insulin is the fattening hormone and that fat doesn't make our bodies produce insulin, whereas carbs do. Our ancestors ate most of their food in the form of fat, as they lived on animals and animal products. So, fat has to be a key part of our diet. In summary, therefore, we need fat, it doesn't make us fat, we have lived on fat for hundreds of years and it performs several vital functions within our bodies.

Q) Are there good fats and bad fats?

A) Yes – the good fats, which we need, are the ones that are found in natural foods, as delivered by nature. The bad fats, which we absolutely do not need, are the ones found in some processed foods, as delivered by food manufacturers. The latter are called trans fats and they are found in margarine, shortening and anywhere where you see the description 'hydrogenated' fats.

Any fats found in real food cannot be bad for us – whether saturated or unsaturated – or humans would have died out, or evolved not to need these foods. There is clearly no evidence of either.

It is also wrong to assume that different foods deliver a single fat. You may be surprised to know that the main fat in pork, beef and eggs is monounsaturated fat – not saturated fat. Fish is not all polyunsaturated fat, as is so often implied. Blue fin Tuna fish, as an example, is 69% protein. Of the 31% that is fat, approximately 30% of this is saturated fat, 37% is monounsaturated fat and 33% is polyunsaturated fat. Olive oil – that well-known 'monounsaturated' fat, is 14% saturated fat. You can check any of this for yourselves on the many nutritional information web sites available to us today – sadly a better source of information than public health advice.

Q) Why do you call fish and lean chicken fat? I've always thought of them as low fat.

A) What a great question. The key things you need to take away from this book are:

- With a couple of exceptions, food is fat/protein or carb/protein, as protein is in everything. Strictly speaking we should describe fish and chicken as fat/protein (they contain zero carbohydrate). We just drop the word protein for simplicity;

- Anything 'from a face' is a fat. When you eat fats (meat, fish, eggs, cheese etc) your body produces no insulin whatsoever and insulin is what makes you fat. Carbs are the things that cause insulin to be produced so we must eat good carbs (so that the body can release the right amount of insulin) and limit how often we eat them.

The answer to the question, therefore, is – even though fish and chicken are lower fat than steak and lamb, they still come from things with faces and therefore they are fats for the purpose of this book. They are fats because they have no impact on insulin. If you eat them at the same time as carbs, your body will use the carbs for energy and store the fat and you don't want this to happen.

Q) Do I need to trim the fat of my meat? (I hope not)

A) No. If you eat meat you are having a fat meal and therefore you can eat meat fat, or any other fat, at the same time. Do you think cave men would have trimmed the fat of meat?! And did you know that lard (pig fat) is more monounsaturated fat than saturated? Fat from real food is not bad for us – shout it from the rooftops.

Q) I like tripe, is that OK? It is lovely with tomatoes on a hot day.

A) Tripe? How can you ask a veggie about tripe?! My carnivore hubby chef told me that tripe is an animal/fat thing so I've looked it up in the dictionary. I laughed – the dictionary definition is "*First or second stomach of e.g. an Ox, as food; slang – worthless or trashy thing, rubbish*". Honest truth – that is what it says. Joking apart, if you tell me tripe is lovely with tomatoes on a hot day then have it. It is a fat, so don't have it with bread, rice or other carbs. If you see a reference in my next book to a fabulous woman who eats tripe it will be you!

The learning for anyone else from this question is the 'face' rule – anything from something with a face is a fat meal. So, kidneys, liver, frogs' legs, snails – all go with fat meals.

Q) Is it OK to eat full fat cheddar cheese? I seem to be eating quite a bit of it, especially if I feel peckish.

A) It is OK to eat full fat cheddar with a fat meal (steak/meat/fish/salad/veg etc). Don't eat cheese with any carbs, as your body will just use the carbs and store the fat. Take care that this is not a dairy Food Intolerance problem. If you can't imagine the day without milk or cheese, start to suspect dairy intolerance pretty quickly.

Protein

Q) Are olives classed as protein or carbs?

A) Don't worry about protein – as it is in everything. The question should be – are olives fats or carbs? The answer is olives are a fat product (as is olive oil). There is barely a trace of carbohydrate in olives. So they can be eaten with fat meals (steak, cheese salad, omelettes, fish etc), but don't have them in large quantities with carb meals (rice, pasta etc). A few with a carb meal won't make much difference – as they are so small.

Q) Pulses: I'm a Vegetarian, but I'm not a big fan of things like Tofu and Quorn and had thought that pulses e.g. mung beans, would be a good substitute for meat? However, your book has pulses and beans listed as carbohydrates. Do they contain both? If so, how can I get some protein in my diet without mixing protein and carbs in one meal and not eating meat or Tofu/Quorn/soya?

A) Pulses (kidney beans, chick peas, lentils, etc) are both carb and protein, not fat/protein, so they are carb meals. Don't be confused with protein. Everything has protein in it – the key foods to separate are carbs and fats.

The kidney bean based veggie chilli recipe in this book is absolutely delicious, if you want to give it a try. Don't worry about not getting enough protein – most people get up to 10 times as much protein as they actually need each day. One tiny slice of cheese or a boiled egg is enough for most people, but we eat half a cow and wonder why we can't move! Bread, rice, cereal etc also all contain protein, so it is in many foods you don't even think of. That's before you have any yoghurt or milk.

Mixing

Q) Could I have cheese with a baked potato, or would I have to eat it separately?

A) Baked potatoes are carbs, so you need to eat low/non fat things with them. You can have low fat cottage cheese, therefore, or ratatouille, or Vegetarian chilli/curry – any low/non fat item.

Q) I'm doing Phase 1 and today I had egg, tomato, onion and brown rice for my breakfast, and then speaking to my friend (who gave me the book and is also following the diet) she said I'm not to mix the egg and rice together. Isn't this just in Phase 2 or have I done it wrong already?

A) You are right and your friend is wrong. In Phase 1 we don't worry about not mixing fats and carbs, as Phase 1 can be quite tough, so we want to make it as easy as possible. Phase 1 also gets the results without adding in this rule from Phase 2. Your breakfast sounds fabulous, so stick with it. The weight loss in Phase 1 is so great that the mixing has no real impact.

Q) Can I eat brown rice with meat?

A) In Phase 1, yes, you can have brown rice with meat. We don't worry about mixing in Phase 1, because it is tough enough already and the weight loss tends to be spectacular, no matter what you eat with what.

In Phase 2, no. Rule 2 says don't mix brown rice with meat because brown rice is a carb and meat is a fat and not mixing the two is one of the best ways to speed up weight loss.

In Phase 3, yes. Rule 2 is the key one that I drop to make sure I don't lose any more weight. This means I can have bread and cheese together (wholemeal cheddar ploughman's) and pasta in cream and cheese sauces, but by staying off processed foods most of the time I don't put on any weight.

Q) How come I can have olive oil with a carb meal?

A) The summary table of fat and carb meals specifically lists "*olive oil for cooking*". If you stir-fry vegetables, as we recommend, the amount of olive oil you end up with, to accompany your brown rice, will be tiny. Dunking wholemeal bread in olive oil is not an option – olive oil is for cooking only with carb meals.

Q) How long should I leave between a fat meal and a carbohydrate meal?

A) The general guideline is three to four hours, because this is how long it normally takes for food to be digested. You should achieve this naturally by having three meals a day. Take care if you are having snacks between meals as you could have a 'fat' snack mid morning and then a carbohydrate meal at lunchtime before the fat snack is out of the way. You will need to allow for snacks in these time guidelines, therefore, and not eat a carb meal within three to four hours of a fat snack, or vice versa.

Q) If fruit were eaten as a snack, would I have to wait three to four hours before eating a fat meal? If I have an apple at 3pm, and want to eat dinner at 5pm, would it have to be a carbohydrate dinner?

A) You're getting into the 'advanced' class with this question. There is a rigid (black and white) answer to this question and there is a flexible (grey) answer to the question. The black and white rules for Phase 2 keep everyone on the right track, but the smart people want to know the shades of grey, so that they can make the diet work perfectly for them.

The black and white answer is – if you have an apple at 3pm, you should have a carb meal at 5pm as this is within three to four hours (and you should have had a carb lunch, or eaten before noon). The black and white answer is ideal if you are planning to have 'rack of lamb' for dinner at 5pm. If, however, you are having fish or chicken or some 'lean' fat at 5pm, then you will be OK having an apple at 3pm. This is because apples are moderate carbs (not bread or potatoes) and fish and chicken are moderate fats (not lamb). So you are not mixing either extreme.

I hope this makes sense – the key thing is to stick to the diet and to get rid of your cravings. If an apple at 3pm and a chicken stir-fry at 5pm helps you do this, that's the way this diet will work for you.

7) Shopping

Q) I am finding it difficult to get Natural Live Yoghurt (NLY) and also wholemeal bread? Should I be going to a health food shop?

A) NLY should be available in main supermarkets, and you will definitely find it in health food shops. It is sometimes called "Bio" yoghurt and sometimes you will just see "active cultures" listed – these are the key words to look for. It has a pretty good shelf life so you can always stock up.

Wholemeal bread – again – you can find in supermarkets but you do have to read every label. Try the organic wholemeal loaves in supermarkets. They tend to have fewer ingredients altogether, so they are much less likely to have sugar and other processed things.

Q) Are sliced cold meats from the deli in the supermarket OK?

A) Sliced meats from the deli are generally OK – you can check with the server that they are cuts from pure cooked meat and that they don't have added sugars or other carbs. Generally it is the packaged hams and meats that have dextrose and sugars added.

Q) I'm finding it difficult to get bacon – all the bacon in supermarkets has preservatives – any tips?

A) Bacon/packaged meats generally are a challenge. Preservatives are actually OK. The key thing to avoid is sugar and all the things with 'ose' – dextrose is the main one they slip into ham and bacon. The bacon over the counter should be just cut meat, or go for any packaged bacon without an 'ose' in it.

Q) I have found a preserve (jam) that does not contain any sugar or artificial ingredients, but it does contain grape extract to sweeten it. As fruit juices are a 'no no' can I have this?

A) Grape extract, as a sweetener, sounds OK. There will be very little grape extract in a small portion of jam, but don't have too much of it, too often.

Q) I have tried to find sugar-free preserve (jam), but have only come across those containing saccharin, is this ok?

A) No – please see the most frequently asked question on sweeteners. You should be able to find sugar-free preserves, without sweeteners, in health food shops. If not, it is very easy to take pure fruit (gooseberries, strawberries or other berries as examples) and to purée it in boiled water on the stove. Add a tiny bit of water to the fruit and keep stirring/simmering until it is all mushy and the water is mostly evaporated off. You can then use this as a spread, or as a natural flavouring for yoghurt.

Q) Is wholemeal couscous the same as the stuff I normally buy in supermarkets?

A) Essentially yes. You can get wholemeal couscous from some health food shops but the normal couscous in supermarkets is absolutely fine as a 'good' carbohydrate.

Q) Is it OK to eat branded sugar-free muesli in Phase 2?

A) Home-made muesli is better than the bought stuff. "*Sugar-free Alpen ®*", as an example, has no added sugar but it is too high in dried fruit sugar for Phase 2. (You can taste the sweetness). If you are a guest at someone's house, sugar-free muesli is better than any sugared cereal, but not as good as porridge.

8) Drinks

Q) What should I drink?

A) Ideally plenty of water, decaffeinated drinks and herbal teas at every phase of the diet.

Phase 1 – water, herbal teas, decaffeinated coffee or tea (no milk).

Phase 2 – water, herbal teas, decaffeinated coffee or tea, milk (if you are tolerant to milk), an occasional glass of wine with the main meal (if you are tolerant to yeast and grapes and Candida is not a problem for you). Also – remember the caffeine exception in Chapter 7 – if you must have a cup of caffeine coffee or tea to start the day then do. The key thing is to stick to the diet.

Phase 3 – what you want, but don't cheat too much, too often and be alert and stay in control.

Q) Can I drink tea with skimmed milk any time of the day in Phase 2?

A) Yes. The quantity of milk added to tea is so small that it will barely register as a carb or a fat. The only people who have to avoid it are those with milk intolerance, but I have actually come across few people with milk intolerance. Don't forget normal tea has caffeine, which raises your blood glucose level and causes insulin to be released, so it is like having a 'cheat.' Stick to decaf tea and you can have several a day, if you really are a tea person.

If this question were about milk in *coffee*, the answer could be different. If you just have a dash of milk in decaf coffee, the answer would be the same and you can drink these without worry throughout the day. Avoid milky coffees (especially large coffee shop lattes), or the milk carb content will soon add up and the body will need to deal with the measurable carb intake each time.

Q) Can I have sugar-free/low cal drinks?

A) Sugar-free/low cal drinks always contain sweeteners (check out the sweetener question) and they may contain caffeine (diet coke/diet Pepsi etc). Caffeine will stimulate the production of insulin, which is the fattening hormone. Sweeteners will keep your taste for sweet things alive and they have no nutritional value, so they are best avoided on a regular basis and kept for occasional 'cheats'.

If you are really determined to have sugar-free drinks in Phase 2, try to limit yourself to no more than one can a day and fill up on water and herbal teas or decaf coffee/tea as much as possible. (Caffeine free diet coke is probably better than the fruit diet drinks, as orange and pineapple type drinks taste even sweeter).

Q) My 17 year old daughter is now on Phase 2, but doesn't like tea/coffee and is getting really fed up with plain water. Is caffeine free coke OK? Or a splash of diluting orange better (or something else)?

A) Caffeine free diet coke has no nutritional value, but I do drink it myself at times, as I also get bored with water. It is OK on occasions therefore. It is obviously best to drink plain water, but it is also important to drink lots, so anything that can help your daughter drink is better than her dehydrating. You can, therefore, add a dash of sugar-free concentrate to water to make it more drinkable (as little as you can get away with to change the taste). You can do this with hot water in the winter (or blackcurrant tea is very similar).

Q) You say that it is better not to drink at all with meals as it affects digestion, I'm finding this quite difficult and just wanted to check that this does include even water? I'm now drinking loads of water throughout the day but miss not having a drink with my meal. (Water that is, not alcohol!)

A) You can drink with meals – it has little to do with weight loss, but it is just a general health tip. Your body digests food more easily when you don't drink anything with meals – even water – because then the natural digestive juices can get to work. If you drink anything with meals, you flood your digestive juices and digestion is made more difficult.

If you never suffer from indigestion, and enjoy drinking with meals, then do. I often have a decaf coffee after meals, or peppermint tea, (which aids digestion), but I rarely drink with meals just because I don't want to water down the taste of the food. My hubby invariably has water with meals, and often red wine, so each to their own.

Q) My only problem is the drinks allowed. I've tried drinking my tea and coffee black, but can't get to like the taste. Could you please tell me if I can have a slice of lemon in a cup of black tea, or in a glass of water, in Phase 1?

A) You only need to do Phase 1 for five days, so milk needs to be avoided for just a short period of time. A slice of lemon in drinks during Phase 1 will be fine. Also try herbal teas – blackcurrant tea is delicious, and camomile and peppermint are two other classics.

Lemon is not great in drinks for dental reasons – the acid, especially when warm, attacks tooth enamel. When I read articles advising people to start the day with a cup of hot water and lemon I worry about the teeth of anyone who follows this advice.

Q) Can I have fruit teas in Phase 1?

A) Yes. All reference to herbal tea includes any fruit, flower or spice varieties: e.g. apple & blackcurrant, lemon & ginger, elderflower, Echinacea, chamomile – these are all great, in whatever quantities you want, at any stage of the diet. Rooibos tea (also known as Rooibosch or red bush tea) is naturally decaffeinated and is also fine. The one to avoid is green tea, as it has measurable caffeine content.

Q) I am 5ft 2in and weigh 215lbs so have a long way to go to get anywhere near my natural weight and there is no way on this earth I can do Phase 2 without drinking, as I go out socially a lot. If I do drink during Phase 2 what do you recommend I stick to? (Red wine is out as it gives me a migraine).

A) Options are dry white wine or low carb beers. Spirits are really bad, as they are so sugary, but you could try one shot of vodka or gin (rum is too sweet) with a large sugar-free tonic or mixer to make a 'long drink'. Another option is to really cut back on the food on social drinking evenings and, in effect, save your cheating for the drink. This would mean having a steak and salad, or Salade Niçoise, or just one simple course and then have more of the dinner in liquid form. Drinking is obviously not as healthy as eating, but I do appreciate that people need to get on with their lives whilst losing weight, so hopefully this may help.

9) Medical Considerations

Q) Do you have any tips for **constipation**?

A) Any change of diet, even to a really healthy way of eating, can upset bowel regularity. Constipation can be greatly helped by the following:

- Drinking as much water, decaf coffee and tea and herbal teas as you can. Constipation is usually due to not having enough liquids, rather than the food being eaten;

- Eating as much salad and veg. as you can – the veggie chilli, butternut squash curry and aubergine recipes in the book are all very filling and they are full of fibre and nutrients;

- Adding fruit back in to your diet – albeit in limited quantities if you have Candida and/or Hypoglycaemia;

- Having more brown rice, rice pasta and porridge oats – you don't have to limit the quantities in Phase 2, so eat what you feel you need;

- The final tip it to find your 'Poo tolerance level of Vitamin C'. (If you take too much Vitamin C, the body will get rid of it in your poo and it can cause loose bowel movements, or even diarrhoea if taken in excessive quantities). This is what nutritionists mean when they talk about the 'poo tolerance level of Vitamin C'. This means taking Vitamin C in quantities just below that which makes you go to the toilet. This is generally seen as the level of Vitamin C that your body can tolerate and, therefore, needs.

Q) Having read *Why do you overeat*? I notice that it seems to be mainly about the production and effects of insulin on fat storage etc. As an insulin dependent **Diabetic**, I was wondering whether your diet would actually work for me?

A) My brother is also an insulin dependent Diabetic, which is how I first started my interest in food, carbs and insulin etc. No doubt you have a doctor assigned to help with your Diabetes, as my brother does. It is really important to work with your doctor, if you do try any change in eating habits, as Diabetes is a serious and delicate illness to manage.

I hope that your doctor is supportive of your weight loss goals, as well as your overall health goals. I also hope that s/he would support a diet advising the consumption of real food and staying away from processed foods. Finally, I hope that your doctor is acutely aware that insulin is the fattening hormone, and that carb and insulin management will be the secret to your weight loss.

You should be able to work with your doctor to reduce your insulin intake over time, by eating a better diet. Before insulin was invented, the only way people could survive Diabetes was by eating a virtually carbohydrate free diet, so that no insulin production was required by the body.

Sadly too many doctors and dieticians give Diabetics the same weight loss advice that they give non-Diabetics i.e. *"base your meals on starchy foods"*. This keeps the Diabetic in a 'high blood glucose/need insulin' state and I am not alone in thinking that this verges on medical malpractice.

The diet could work well for you, but you will need to find a doctor that shares similar views and work with them on your weight loss goals, as Diabetes is such a critical condition.

Q) Can I do The Harcombe Diet whilst **pregnant**?

A) Yes. This is the only diet that I would recommend for someone who is pregnant. Here are three top tips for pregnant women who want to lose weight and/or not gain too much during pregnancy:

1) Don't eat less; eat better. Eat only real food – meat, fish, eggs, dairy products, salads, vegetables, fruits and whole grains (e.g. brown rice, porridge oats) – nothing processed (obviously follow all the extra pregnancy advice about avoiding pate, raw eggs and soft cheese etc). You and baby-to-be will be much better off without trans fats and sugars and you will find real food naturally fills you up, without blood sugar highs and lows and the cravings that go with this roller coaster. Try to limit even the good carbs you eat – insulin resistance develops in pregnant women (and leads to diabetes in 2-4% of cases) and only carbs cause insulin to be needed/released.

2) Eat regularly. Go for three substantial meals a day, based around meat, fish, eggs and dairy and with large portions of salads & vegetables (limit, or avoid, potatoes, as these are high carb). If you must snack, go for lower sugar fruits, like apples or pears. A key goal during pregnancy should be to keep your blood glucose level nice and stable and keep any sweet cravings at bay.

3) Don't eat more than you need. Many women wrongly believe that they need to eat for two - a woman actually needs no more energy (calories) in the first trimester and barely 300 calories a day more than normal in the final stage of pregnancy. That amounts to 75g of dry porridge oats made with water, not milk. The average baby only weighs about 7-8 lbs at birth, and the fluids around it add up to not much more than a stone, so there is no need to put on more than a couple of stone during pregnancy.

Q) I have been diagnosed as having elevated insulin – otherwise known as **Syndrome X** or **Insulin Resistance**. Is this the same as Hypoglycaemia?

A) Hypoglycaemia, Syndrome X and Insulin Resistance do have a relationship. Let's try to put this as simply as possible…

Hypoglycaemia is a medical term for low blood sugar. It is often seen as the 'opposite' of Diabetes, as people with Diabetes have sugar in their blood (and urine) and yet someone in a state of Hypoglycaemia has low glucose in their blood and may therefore be experiencing light headedness, shaky hands, irritability and all the other symptoms of a low blood glucose level.

Hypoglycaemia is often seen as a sign that the pancreas has pumped out too much insulin when carbohydrates have been eaten. (You drink apple juice, your body thinks you have eaten 20 apples and so releases the amount of insulin to 'mop up' the 20 apples and your blood glucose level actually ends up lower than before you drank the juice). This condition is sometimes seen as the pancreas working 'too well', but it is often the slippery slope to the pancreas starting to not work well at all – this brings us to:

Insulin resistance. This describes the situation where our bodies don't respond properly to the release of insulin. With insulin resistance, eating carbohydrates causes insulin to be released, but the body fails to use this insulin efficiently and, therefore, the carbohydrates get stored as more fat instead, adding to your weight problem further. It has been shown that 92% of people with Type II Diabetes have insulin resistance. (Type II Diabetes is the one developed by older people – not the one that teenagers tend to get very suddenly). It is hoped that, by identifying the signs as early as possible, people may be able to change their eating patterns to avoid serious health problems in the future.

Syndrome X is a term used by doctors to group together a number of conditions, which they have often seen together in a patient. They have observed that people with insulin resistance are also highly likely to have: insulin resistance; raised blood fats; raised cholesterol; raised blood glucose levels; high blood pressure and so on. By looking at these conditions together they are able to treat the patient 'holistically' and try to address all the problems together as they are linked – all related to the weight and blood glucose handling mechanism of the patient.

Q) Are there any other Phase 1 breakfast options for someone **allergic to eggs**?

A) Here are some breakfast options for anyone allergic to eggs:

1) Fish: This does seem a bit strange, but Haddock is quite a normal breakfast dish, apparently;

2) Natural Live Yoghurt;

3) Bacon, on its own;

4) Brown rice cereal, instead of the brown rice allowance.

5) Flexing outside the rules a bit, another cereal option is porridge oats – 100% whole porridge oats with nothing added. Go for the regular size oats, not jumbo ones, as they mix more easily. Because you shouldn't have milk in Phase 1 you can just pour boiling water straight onto the oats, stir and eat. It is hugely filling and a great way to start the day. Swap porridge oats, gram for gram, with the brown rice allowance. So 50g of porridge oats (before the water is poured on) replaces the whole meat/fish

eater rice allowance and Vegetarians can have 75g of porridge oats, to replace 75g of rice, for example.

This is not strictly within the rules of Phase 1, but porridge is rarely a food to which people are intolerant and, if it helps someone get off to a great start with Phase 1, it is worth the flexibility. (People who are not allergic to eggs may also like to try this if they are struggling with Phase 1 breakfast options).

10) Personal questions

Q) Over the last four years, I have been putting on weight, regardless of the fact that I am definitely not eating as many calories as most "*normal*" people. I read your book and understood how my metabolism should be shot. I am writing to you as I hope with your research and experience you may be able to tell me if this is normal for people with eating disorders and the best way to sort out the metabolism. (This reader shared lots more info in the email, so I've just shared the headlines of the query and the bits of my reply that I think may be of general benefit to other readers).

A) On the weight gain, this must feel awful – especially when it seems unrelated to the food that you are eating. Here are a few thoughts:

- I would recommend seeing your doctor just so that an under active thyroid can be ruled out (this can be tested with a blood test and unexplained weight gain and extreme tiredness are two of the most common symptoms). I wouldn't place too much hope on this being an explanation as it is quite rare (it is not a nice condition anyway, so I hope you don't have this).

- Please don't be offended by this, but you may be eating more than you think. I kept a food diary for a brief time during my research and I was quite surprised at all the things I 'grazed' on during the day. Keeping a food diary for a week or two could help identify patterns (and would almost certainly help you identify any Food Intolerances).

- You do sound like a classic candidate for the advice in the book. A low fat diet is a high carb diet, as hopefully the book has explained. Everything in your note says that all of the three conditions could be problems for you and, something like wheat intolerance, can cause people to gain pounds – sometimes almost overnight – as the body holds water for some reason when it consumes a food to which it is intolerant. Have you tried Phase 1? Has this helped? I would be surprised if it didn't.

Q) My eyesight has improved – is this related to the change in diet?

A) Quite likely. This is not surprising and I have seen it with other case studies. It is a well-known fact that Diabetics are at great risk of eye problems, e.g. glaucoma. Diabetics tend to have sugar in their blood constantly, as they have no insulin naturally available to mop up the sugar (they inject, or take tablets instead). So, cutting out sugar has reduced the level of sugar in your body and has made your body less like a simulator for a Diabetic. It follows that this would help your eyesight. Yet another benefit of eating real food.

Q) I am trying to have a baby. Common sense tells me this diet is healthier than my 'Sir Scoffs-a-lot' diet before, but if I am fortunate enough to conceive what will happen? Will I continue to 'naturally' dispose of UNnecessary body fat? Even allowing for a pregnant lady there is still a good 2 stone of excess fat adhered to various bits of my anatomy! Obviously at some point I will put weight on (as you do with another person inside you) but that is not usually for a good 2/3 months. Any ideas?

A) Congratulations to be! This is such a healthy diet it will be great for someone planning to get pregnant, or actually pregnant. People should not try to eat less in either of these situations, so eating the right things, rather than trying to eat less, will be a good thing to do. The avoidance of processed foods will also help a lot during pregnancy, as temporary Diabetes is a common problem for pregnant women, as their blood glucose level goes haywire with the baby. For some women the Diabetes is not temporary, which must be horrendous – you end up with a baby and Diabetes for life.

Most doctors advise women to lose weight before getting pregnant, but you don't have masses to lose and you are not cutting calories so you should be fine. Often weight loss helps women get pregnant too (the body just generally functions better at its correct weight), which, I guess, is why they advise women to lose weight first. Hopefully you will be feeling great, eating healthy foods, and things will happen naturally at the right time. You will be doing yourself a lot of favours by zapping Candida and Food Intolerances before getting pregnant, as both can develop/worsen during pregnancy.

You should continue to lose your excess body weight, as you eat healthy foods and nourish your body. You may well lose a stone before getting pregnant and then continue to lose before the baby really starts growing. The average baby only weighs about 7-8lb at birth, and the fluids around it add up to not much more than a stone, so there is no need to put on more than a couple of stone during pregnancy. If you continue to eat no processed foods and lots of healthy foods you should find that you don't have too much to lose afterwards.

Q) My wife and I are following the principles as laid down in your book but are finding that, whereas we both lost weight in Phase 1, we are stuck whilst following Phase 2. Is this normal? I have only been on Phase 2 for a week so I may be expecting too much but my wife has been on it longer and her weight loss has all but stopped.

We are following the rules religiously and are finding that cravings have ceased and hunger is minimised. So there has been some good! I would appreciate your advice.

A) The first thing I check is that people are following the rules, but you are so we can discount this one (the most common mistake is people snacking too much and/or having carb snacks too close to a fat meal, or vice versa).

I have observed this 'plateau' in weight loss with a number of people. For some it happens quite soon into Phase 2, and for others quite a bit later. Where it happens quite soon, I have observed that it seems to take the body some time to adjust to getting fuel from real food rather than from processed foods. Sugar, white rice, white flour etc are much easier for the body to get energy from (despite the fact that it is non nutritious energy) and I am seeing quite a few cases where bodies are taking some time to adjust to getting energy efficiently from real food.

It is as if our bodies have become lazy and they need to re-learn how to work properly with real food. In the cases where people have plateaued, early in Phase 2, this has passed within 1-4 weeks (4 was the longest I have seen and this has only happened with one person) and then weight loss has been steady thereafter.

Another thing you may want to try is staying off wheat for the first few weeks in Phase 2. I have yet to work with someone for whom wheat has **not** been a problem. The weight loss, when wheat is avoided, confirms that wheat has been a problem.

Try porridge or 100% puffed rice cereal for breakfast (or egg and bacon) instead of shredded wheat or wheat based muesli. Get rice pasta, instead of wheat pasta, (you can get this in supermarkets now, not just health food shops) for eating with the 15 minute tomato sauce and stay off whole wheat bread at the same time. You may well find that you both have wheat intolerance and this is making the body hold water and impacting weight loss. The good news is that this will ease when your immune system is strong and healthy so you will be able to return to wheat in time.

The final bit of good news is that everyone I have worked with, and those who email me, all say that a pound lost on this diet stays off. Because you have not calorie counted, you have not slowed your metabolism down and you are actually boosting your immune system rather than weakening it. So, if you lose a few pounds and then plateau and then lose a few more, you will get there and you will know that you are doing your body and energy a whole heap of good in the process.

Q) I have noticed that I get into 'virtuous' and 'vicious' circles. I start eating healthily and it goes well for a few days. Then I have something I shouldn't and the cravings come back – why is this?

A) It sounds like this is a classic case of cheating too much too soon. You need to do Phase 1 and then stick with Phase 2 for some time, before your immune system is back in good shape and then you will be able to get away with a bit of cheating. What is actually going on is related to the three conditions:

<u>Hypoglycaemia</u>

After eating the craved food your blood glucose level, which has been quite stable for days, is suddenly jolted back into the peaks and troughs of Hypoglycaemia. Your blood glucose level rises quickly and gives you a huge high that you may not have had for days. This, however, is then followed by the big trough as your body releases (too much) insulin and your blood glucose level drops lower than it was before. Then the cravings come back big time. Your blood glucose level is so low that your body cries out for any carbohydrate – just to raise your blood glucose level again. That one bit of processed food suddenly leads to more processed foods and you are into a full-scale binge.

Food Intolerance

Having stayed off your trigger foods for a few days, you could have a number of reactions after suddenly eating a food to which you are intolerant. A few people experience quite violent and unpleasant symptoms as the body sensibly alerts you to the fact that this is an unwelcome food.

In *Not all in the Mind* by Dr Richard Mackarness, a situation is described whereby a man, badly intolerant to eggs, avoided them for a period of time and then ate them in a cake without realising and literally collapsed after eating them.

You may find, if you are quite intolerant to wheat, for example, that you experience quite strong symptoms after eating wheat for the first time in a few days. Symptoms can include severe bloating, an 'upset' stomach, significant water retention (illustrated by the fact that some people can weigh up to 7lb heavier from one day to the next when they eat a food to which they are intolerant) and a general feeling of being unwell.

Other people can feel 'elation' after returning to their addictive substances and they are immediately caught back in the trap of cravings and food addiction. They may still have adverse reactions (water retention is one of the most common) but there is also a psychological wellbeing, which makes it difficult to continue to avoid the offending food(s). Whether you experience positive feelings, or just negative reactions, you will have re-introduced your 'poison' to your body and the cravings will start to return. In Chapter 8, on weight maintenance, where we talk about 'cheating', you will note that you need to be very sensitive to your own susceptibility to cravings.

Candida

The third thing that happens when you eat a food, which you have avoided for some time, is that you may reawaken the Candida overgrowth inside you, which you are unlikely to have killed off with just a few days healthy eating. As soon as you eat yeasty and sugary foods you start to feed the Candida again and your Candida led cravings will rapidly return.

In as little as one day, and certainly in no more than three to five days, you can move from a virtuous circle to a vicious circle. The good news is that you can break out of a vicious circle to a virtuous circle in the same amount of time.

You need to get your immune system strong again, free from Candida and Food Intolerance and your blood glucose well under control before you can start to cheat. At the moment, when you can move so quickly from a virtuous circle to a vicious circle, this is a clear indication that your immune system is not strong enough and you need to be free from Candida, Food Intolerance and Hypoglycaemia before you try to cheat. Don't lose heart. You will be able to cheat and there is nothing like savouring the taste of dark chocolate when you **want** to eat it rather than when you **need** to.

Q) I was so excited by your book! I started a month and a half ago just before my holiday and stuck to it all week. I have now been happy with no cravings and in control (I believe I suffer from Hypoglycaemia, as I had huge cravings for bread, cereal, chocolate and would binge till sick) but I haven't lost any weight. I am eating so well I just don't understand how I can go from binging and eating so much sugar and refined products to eating healthily and no weight change. I am getting so tired of feeling trapped in a fat me, any suggestions welcome?

A) I think you've got all three conditions going on. Cravings for bread, cereal and chocolate could well be wheat and sugar intolerance, as well as Hypoglycaemia, and you have almost certainly fed your Candida with all the binge eating and starvation (your immune system must be in a heck of a state).

I have seen quite a few case studies like you who have mucked up their metabolisms and sugar handling mechanisms so much that there is not an immediate result when they start a healthy diet like this one. However, every one of them has lost weight when they have stuck at it. I had one case study that lost just one pound the first time she did Phase 1 and then nine pounds when she repeated it again a few weeks later. I don't understand everything about our bodies, but I do observe some of them taking some time to realise that something new and good is happening.

I would advise the following:

- Don't give up – you should be hugely heartened by the fact that you know how to ditch those cravings. Life without cravings is just so liberating;

- Just think – we are heading into the woolly jumper season and if you lose just one pound a week you will emerge in the spring at least 20 pounds lighter (this email arrived in autumn);

- Put all your effort into keeping the cravings away and the weight loss will follow. I would recommend doing Phase 1 once a month, just to keep the three conditions at bay. I would advise keeping off wheat for a few weeks in Phase 2 (have rice pasta instead of wheat pasta and baked potatoes instead of bread). Keep fruit to just 1-2 portions a day to make sure that Candida stays away and eat as much salad and vegetables as you can manage to fill up with fibre and nutrients;

- Finally – do everything you can to rebuild your immune system and to be nice to yourself instead of being horrid:

- Take a multi vitamin/mineral every day (this also makes sure you avoid any strange cravings that happen when you miss a key nutrient);

- Get a pedometer and start upping your step rate – even just a 10 minute walk each day – in case your metabolism is particularly sluggish;

- Get as much daylight as you can during the winter and try to do something every day that you enjoy just for you;

- The bottom line is that you've got to start being nice to yourself – you wouldn't stuff and starve your best friend, so don't do it to yourself. Put the energy you have previously put into stuffing and starving into nourishing.

Q) I looked up 'Biotin' as you say it inhibits Candida. I understand it is found in mushrooms, watermelon, strawberries, peanuts and yeast. All these are banned on the five-day anti-Candida diet. Can you explain as I would have thought one should eat more Biotin to inhibit Candida rather than less?

A) Wow – you're getting into the advanced class. Well done for starting your own research, as this makes looking after your own health so much more interesting and productive.

The answer is that Biotin is a vitamin that is useful to attack Candida, but it is best taken in vitamin tablet form (or in liver, kidneys and egg yolks which are other good sources).

Biotin can be found in all the foods that you mention but these foods also have yeast, fruit sugars, moulds and other things that feed the Candida, so the disadvantages are more than outweighed by the traces of the Biotin that they contain.

Hence stick to the tablets, or eggs and animal organs, and leave the other foods until the Candida has been zapped.

Q) I'm on the first day of Phase 2. Feeling very proud of myself for getting through Phase 1 and I've lost 6 lbs. I've suffered from terrible indigestion for years and during the five days of Phase 1, I haven't had any problems at all.

I was convinced I had Candida, as I've had terrible sugar cravings, but I've just had a bowl of porridge and my indigestion has come back with a vengeance. Does this mean I might have Food Intolerance, rather than Candida, or possibly both?

A) You could have all three conditions going on, but the two that could cause indigestion after porridge are Food Intolerance and Candida.

If you had a high score on the Candida questionnaire, this will not have been cured during Phase 1, although it does get severely attacked during the first five days. To kill off a bad case of Candida you will need to stick to the three pronged attack (starve it with diet, kill it with medication and keep the causal factors like antibiotics, hormone tablets, stress etc at bay).

To keep up the diet attack you will need to have no more than 1-2 pieces of fruit a day and keep all carbs fairly low (even good carbs can feed the parasite). Go for two fat meals a day therefore. Eat lots of garlic and Natural Live Yoghurt to attack the yeast. Taking vitamins (Biotin etc) will also help.

You may also have Food Intolerance – it is normal to have more than one condition, as they 'feed' each other. Porridge is actually in the wheat family, so you could be intolerant to wheat. You would be quite badly intolerant to wheat if you react to porridge, as it is quite a distant 'relative' in this food family. I still can't have wheat regularly, but I have porridge every day with no problems at all. If you had water with the porridge then you only have the oats to suspect. If you had milk too, then suspect a dairy intolerance, which can give really bad indigestion. Think back – has milk/cheese in the past given you the same problems? Or has it been pasta/pizza/bread – which would be wheat.

I would highly recommend keeping a food diary for a while and noting what you eat, when and then any reaction and the time it occurs. Within a week or two of doing this, when I was doing my research, I could see a crystal clear pattern between what I ate and what was causing me problems. Eat just one food at each meal for a while or eat something you suspect (a slice of bread) with foods that you know are OK (veg/salad etc).

Q) After reading your book, I have two of the conditions (Food Intolerance and Hypoglycaemia) and am treating them as advised in your book. The only thing I am worried about is what to do each month, as in previous attempts on any diet/change of eating plan, my efforts have always been sabotaged two weeks before my period with the unbelievable cravings for refined food, especially bucket-fulls of chocolate.

Please can you advise me if there is anything different I need to do two weeks before my period, and during my period, to combat any cravings because I get hit badly with bad fluctuations of low blood sugar?

A) I suffer from cravings at the time of the month as well. Not quite for two weeks though – that is half the month so we need to sort this out. There are a number of things that you can do:

1) Make sure you are taking a good multi vitamin and mineral pill every day. At the back of the book I have included the latest European Recommended Daily Allowances (RDA's) so you can take this to Chemists, Drug Store or the local health food shop and get a good all round tablet.

2) You may like to take one vitamin and one mineral in higher doses, in addition to the daily multi vitamin and mineral. Try taking these just for the two weeks before each period, or every day if you remember and you notice a difference:

a) The vitamin is a good quality multi B vitamin complex. I take one (not every day, but before my period and whenever else I remember) that has approximately 25mg of B6 and then the tablet automatically works out how much of the other B vitamins you need to balance this. If you go to a good health food shop, the staff will be able to advise you on a good multi B complex. The B vitamins are the mood vitamins, so you should also find that PMT symptoms of mood swings, feeling blue, sadness etc all get better.

b) The mineral is chromium – this is the mineral that specifically affects blood glucose levels. There is no European RDA for this, but 200μg is highly recommended and some people have found this alone has a fantastic impact on their sugar/processed carb cravings. Again – a good health store will help you pick one of these.

3) Onto food tips – because you know that the cravings are going to arrive and when – there are several things that you can try:

a) Make sure you start the day with a slow release carb breakfast – porridge (with water or skimmed milk) every day for a week or two before the period will really help fill you up until lunch;

b) Play around with what works for you and increase your number of carb meals during the pre-period time. If I have carb cravings and have an omelette for lunch I find this does nothing to satisfy the cravings. If I have rice pasta with tomato sauce or veggie chilli with brown rice, I find this satisfies me a lot more;

c) Chocolate cravings are often a sign of iron deficiency (and this gets worse around the period itself when we lose blood) so the vitamin tablet will help. You can also do some managed 'cheating' to ease the craving, but only with real chocolate. Allow yourself some chocolate, which must be at least 70% cocoa (ideally 85%, or more). You will find that a square or two of real chocolate will satisfy a chocolate craving much more than sugary confectionery bars. If you have a square or two after both main meals this will still be much better than giving in to cravings for high sugar 'chocolate'. Dark chocolate is an acquired taste so, if you've not had it before, stick with it. Once you get there you will never eat cheap chocolate again.

Q) I could do with some help! I've four children aged 10, 11, 13 and 14yrs and they love things like Spaghetti Bolognese, Lasagne, chilli con carni... do you have any suggestions for cooking for the whole family on Phase 2? I'm really enjoying all the salads, but already they are saying *"not salad again mum!"*

A) The children will be a lot healthier too for cutting out processed foods, so, if you can get them on the brown rice and brown pasta too, you will be doing them a lot of favours. Assuming they don't need to lose weight, they can mix fat and carbs all they like. It only has to be you keeping them separate. So you can:

- Make the 15 minute tomato sauce in the book and pour this on your whole wheat pasta (or rice pasta, if wheat is a problem for you) and the family can have a bolognaise sauce instead. It does mean two pans on the stove, but you can make enough tomato sauce for a couple of nights;

- The veggie chilli recipe in the book is great – you can all eat this together, or make a meat version for them and a non meat (i.e. non fat) version for you. It does take a bit of effort, sadly, but hopefully the weight loss will be worth it;

- Any meat/fish meals with any vegetables are great for you and the children can have rice, pasta or potatoes with the meat/fish/veg/salad – you can give the carbs a miss;

- A great quick meal is baked potatoes – with chilli or tuna bake for them and with low fat cottage cheese or tomato sauce or ratatouille for you;

- You can also make a veggie lasagne for the whole family – use whole wheat or rice pasta strips with loads of vegetables and pour the cheese sauce over 2/3 of the dish only, leaving a fat free bit for you.

Q) I just can't get my fiancé to eat vegetables – please can you help?

A) Here are a few suggestions from the Harcombe man of the household – the chef:

1) The butternut squash curry was a massive hit with our neighbour who similarly hates veg. (You can even blend it just to have a curry sauce and he won't even know there are vegetables in there);

2) Hubby recommends using spicy olive oils for stir-frying peppers, garlic and onions. You can then add strips of beef or chicken to a stir-fry or serve the fried veg with a huge slab of lamb or steak;

3) Most men like cole slaw – you can shred/finely chop carrots, cabbage, celeriac, onions etc and make real mayonnaise (recipe in Part 7) – make it as creamy as you like and serve with fish or meat as a fat meal;

4) Slip a few mushrooms, with cheese and/or ham, into an omelette;

5) Try doing vegetables on a BBQ – aubergine/eggplant, peppers, onions and courgettes, on a skewer, taste fantastic;

6) See if your fiancé will eat salad (experiment with a variety of lettuce leaves and olive oil/balsamic). This will always be a great alternative to vegetables;

7) Finally, the 15 minute tomato sauce is a great source of olive oil and tomatoes – which at least give some good nutrients in vegetable/fruit form.

Q) I start work at 7.00am at the latest and therefore normally eat my breakfast at work (Melon and Strawberries or Cereal). Do you have any ideas for 'packed' breakfasts, especially for Phase 1?

A) If you're really struggling in Phase 1, be a little bit flexible and have plain porridge and water for breakfast. I haven't met anyone intolerant to porridge oats yet, so it is unlikely to cause a problem, or affect weight loss.

Similarly, you could have 100% rice cereal in Phase 1 instead of your rice allowance for the day (or as part of your allowance, if you are Vegetarian). This used to be available only in health food shops but it is now available in supermarkets in the gluten free sections.

Other Phase 1 options are hard-boiled eggs or a tin of tuna. Sounds bizarre, but it really does keep hunger away until lunchtime.

Q) Can you give me a diet plan for the first five days of Phase 1? I am very busy and need this help, I am a theatre sister.

A) I designed a Phase 1 plan for this reader and it is now the "*Planner*" menu for Phase 1 in this book. Here are some other tips for busy people doing The Harcombe Diet:

- Snack on (small) pots of Natural Live Yoghurt, hard-boiled eggs and crudités (chopped carrots, celery sticks etc);

- Don't worry about how often you have the same meals in Phase 1, as it is so short. Stick to a bought pack of salad with a tin of tuna thrown on top or with chicken leftovers, to have quick and simple meals;

- I recommend roasting a chicken and hard-boiling some eggs the day before starting Phase 1 and then you will have good options for meals for a few days;

- Omelettes are also great, as they take fewer than 10 minutes to knock up;

- A Phase 2 tip is to have rice pasta (available in supermarkets as well as health food shops) instead of normal rice, as rice pasta takes about 10 minutes to cook and brown rice about 25 minutes.

Q) I'm a bloke, I don't have an eating disorder and I'm not really overweight. Can I just adopt the rules loosely (i.e. mix carbs and fat at some meals) – I've just got about 4 kilos to lose?

A) Men just love this diet. I'll do a separate book just for men one day, which will be about six pages long. Men don't miss fruit as much as women and they love being able to have steak and pasta – just not at the same time. They love the flexibility with coffee and red wine and they don't seem to mind Phase 1.

You can adopt the rules loosely, however, I would recommend doing Phase 1, even if you've never had eating problems a) because you will lose most of your four kilos during these five days (trust me!) and b) because it really does zap all cravings on the head and it jolts your body into a new way of eating.

I would then recommend having fat meals or carb meals (i.e. **not** mixing) until you lose all the weight you want to (this will be a max of 2-3 weeks). This will help reinforce the fat meal/carb meal concept and you can always go back to this technique whenever you want to lose a bit of weight again.

You will get to Phase 3 in no time and **then** you can adopt the rules loosely and cheat as much as you can get away with. The top 10 tips for cheating are all you need to know. Stick to those and the weight will not go back on. One of my case studies has beer with carb meals and wine with fat meals and he has not put the weight back on. Another has chocolate and mocca frappuccinos in Starbucks ®, but he makes that his lunch and he's not put any of his 28-pound loss back on. Just never waste your cheating.

Q) We started Phase 1 on Wed 28th April it is now 9th May and we have lost quite well. "A" who has never had to diet shed 7lbs and I, who have dieted almost all of my life, managed 11 Pounds. How long is it safe to continue Phase 1? Would it be better to change to Phase 2?

A) You can continue with Phase 1 for as long as you like. Your weight loss suggests that at least one of the conditions has been a problem for you. So, you may want to watch your carbohydrate intake on Phase 2 just to make sure that you keep Candida away and keep your blood glucose stable. I would therefore advise going on to a 'modified' Phase 2. Have just two pieces of fruit a day from the lower sugar fruits list. I would also stay off wheat for a while longer, as I have yet to work with a case study that has not had wheat intolerance.

Q) I started Phase one on Monday it is only Friday tea-time and I have lost 8lbs – I am absolutely delighted! I am heading off to Mexico in a couple of week's time – is it safe enough to go through another 5 days of Phase 1? Would the weight loss be roughly the same?

A) Yes, it is fine to continue with Phase 1 and this is the fastest weight loss stage of the diet so I can see why you may want to stick with this until your holiday.

Sadly you are unlikely to lose another 8lbs in five days, as the closer you get to your goal weight, the slower weight loss gets. Candida and Food Intolerance cause significant water retention, so a lot of the early loss is water, but then your body is approximately 50% water anyway so we should expect to lose both water and fat as we lose weight. It all makes a difference and you should notice your rings and clothes fit better and places like inside thighs are slimmer, as water is often stored here. You should lose another few pounds, though, which will get you close to a stone weight loss in two weeks – not bad just before a holiday.

The next best news is that you can lose another few pounds whilst in Mexico, with hardly any deprivation at all. Just keep the three rules of Phase 2 in your head and have a fat or carb breakfast (this will be either bacon/omelette etc or tropical fruits and sugar-free cereals) and then fat or carb main meals. Most holiday and hotel restaurants are full of seafood and meat/fish dishes with an abundance of salads and vegetables as main meals – just don't have any bread/potatoes/corn chips or any carbs with this meal.

Your carb meal options will be limited – the staple carbs in Mexico are corn and wheat, as they use corn chips, tortillas, taco shells etc. These are all processed carbs and you are unlikely to get wholemeal carbs in Mexico. If you want a carb meal, therefore, go for the veggie tortillas and then you are at least just having carbs and no fat. Or, have taco shells with refried beans and other vegetables. The short hand is carb meal = Vegetarian and fat meal = carnivore. You will be able to try all the great food on offer, therefore, but just don't eat the carbs and the fats at the same time.

Q) Don't laugh because this is a serious question – how do you *stop* losing weight in Phase 3?

A) Wow! Some questions floor me. I had not expected anyone to have this problem, as The Harcombe Diet should help you reach your natural weight. The first thought that springs to mind therefore is – are you sure you are at your natural weight? It could be that you have got used to being at a higher weight for so long that you can't believe this is you.

If you really don't want to lose any more weight, then the best tip is to drop Rule 2 from Phase 2. This means that you can have cheese sandwiches or meat and potatoes, as examples. When you mix the fat and carbs, your body will take the energy it needs from the carbs first and store the fat but if you keep your overall energy need at the right level (enough energy/calories to fuel your daily activity), this won't be a problem. I would always recommend sticking to Rule 1 and would hope that you will never go back to white rice, bread and pasta when the wholemeal alternatives are so much tastier and healthier. Rule 3 is a good idea to stick to also – don't eat the foods that are causing any of your Candida, Food Intolerance and Hypoglycaemia problems.

Q)So what happens now?

A) Here are some final tips for an inspirational boost. It's then over to you – go for it!

You now know why you've struggled to stick to a diet and why you have had food cravings. You have these cravings because of one thing that you are doing, calorie counting, and because of one, or all, of three conditions that you may have – Candida, Food Intolerance and Hypoglycaemia. All of these are closely linked together and they are also linked to and caused by stress, modern medication and modern processed foods.

Calorie counting directly causes cravings, as your body will tell you to give it the energy (calories) that it needs. Candida drives you to crave sugary, yeasty and vinegary foods. Food Intolerance drives you to crave any food to which you are intolerant – this can literally be any food or drink from eggs to alcohol. Hypoglycaemia drives you to crave processed carbohydrates as your blood glucose level lurches from high to low on an hourly basis.

The key to overcoming overeating is to overcome cravings. You have failed so many times before because of these cravings. Stop counting calories; follow the strategies in this book to overcome Candida, Food Intolerance and Hypoglycaemia and you can free yourself from food cravings. When you are free from food cravings you will have a choice as to what you want to eat and when you want to eat it. Right now you do not have that choice – you are not greedy or weak-willed. You are a food addict and you need to go 'cold turkey' on some foods just like a drug addict needs to go 'cold turkey' on their addictive substance.

You will succeed this time because you now have the power of knowledge. You know why you have failed before – because of the cravings. You know what you have been craving and why. You know that the cravings have come from calorie counting, Candida, Food Intolerance and Hypoglycaemia. You know that you have to eliminate the offending foods from your diet and watch the cravings disappear in literally days. You also know not to starve yourself, or to let yourself go hungry, as this is the surest way to slip up in the future.

This is the good news. The bad news is that there are now no excuses. You know why you overeat. You know how to stop it. You know that the only person who can control your eating is you. If you really do want to be slim for life then put all the willpower you undoubtedly do have into fighting food cravings. It won't be easy but nothing worth having ever is. Furthermore, I can promise you two things:

1) It will be worth it. Your health is the most important thing that you have in life – without it you have nothing. You must nurture, nourish and treat your body well rather than starve and stuff it and make yourself ill.

2) It will be easier than you think. You cannot imagine life without certain foods right now because you are addicted to them. In as few as five days, however, you could dramatically reduce that addiction. Every day that you nourish your body and avoid the foods that are harming it is another day nearer the healthy, slim you.

I know how it feels to be where you are now and I know how it feels to be where I am now. I would love every unhappy, overweight, food addict to be happy, slim and healthy and to be able to get on with something infinitely more important than food – life!

I wish you the very best in your journey and I will leave you with some thoughts that I sincerely hope will inspire you along the way:

Q) WHO is going to change your life?

A) You are. It's up to you.

Q) WHEN are you going to change your life?

A) Now! Unless you plan to be overweight for your entire life you've got to start sometime, so do it now. Every day that you continue to feed your food addiction it gets worse. The longer you leave this the harder it gets, so do it now.

Q) HOW will you change your life?

A) By stopping food cravings, because it is cravings that make you overeat when all you want is to be slim.

Q) WHY are you going to change your life?

A) Because you only have one life. You don't intend to waste another day overweight and addicted to food.

Part 7

Recipes

Next to the title of each recipe we have put a few symbols to give you further help 'at a glance':

- ⧖ is an egg timer – for recipes that take fewer than 30 minutes from getting the ingredients out of the fridge/cupboards to sitting down and eating. Some dishes are very quick to prepare but they don't have this symbol because of chilling or marinating time, for example.

- ☺ Is a smiley face – for recipes that are particularly good for children.

- ☺ Is a thumbs up – for recipes for entertaining or special occasions.

The table, at the end of each recipe, shows which phase the recipe is suitable for. Whether it is a carb or a fat meal.

V means suitable for Vegetarians.

C means suitable if you have Candida.

H means suitable if you have Hypoglycaemia.

The two main Food Intolerances are then noted – wheat-free and dairy-free.

The Harcombe Diet Recipe book is all laid out in this format for your convenience.

Phase	Meal	V	C	H	Wheat-free	Dairy-free
1 & 2	Carb	✓	✓	✓	✓	✓

Recipes

The following recipes are in Part 7:

293

- 15 minute tomato sauce
- Aubergine Boats
- Butternut Squash Curry
- Cheese Sauce (for cauliflower cheese or cheesy leeks)
- Char Grilled Vegetables/Vegetable kebabs
- Chef's Salad
- Egg & Asparagus bake
- Four Cheese Salad
- Fruit Platters
- Omelettes (no milk/Phase 1 version);
- Paella (Seafood or Bean)
- Ratatouille
- Roasted Vegetables with Pine Nuts & Parmesan
- Roast Chicken with Garlic & Lemon
- Roast Leg of Lamb with Rosemary & Vegetables
- Salade Niçoise/Salmon Niçoise
- Scrambled eggs (no milk/Phase 1 version);
- Stir-Fry Vegetables
- Stuffed Peppers/Tomatoes
- Vegetarian Chilli

15 Minute Tomato Sauce ✂

This is such a versatile sauce. It goes with pasta, spaghetti, quinoa, Quorn, vegetables and Tofu, or just about anything else you can think of.

Ingredients:

2 tablespoons olive oil 1 onion, finely chopped 1 clove garlic, crushed	400g tin chopped tomatoes 2 teaspoons of basil (ideally fresh) Salt & ground black pepper

Method:

1) Heat the olive oil in a wok, or large frying pan, until it is sizzling.

2) Fry the onion and garlic until soft (2-3 minutes) and then add the chopped tomatoes. These will take approximately 2 minutes to warm through.

3) Add the basil, salt & pepper and you can then serve immediately or leave the sauce to simmer until some pasta is cooked (10-15 minutes).

TIP 1 – To make this a hot and spicy pasta sauce just buy some spicy olive oil and use this for cooking instead. Or, add a finely chopped chilli.

Serves 2

Phase	Meal	V	C	H	Wheat-free	Dairy-free
1 & 2	Either	✓	✓	✓	✓	✓

Aubergine Boats ♻

These look fabulous – definitely impressive enough for a dinner party. Each person gets one boat and they can be served on a bed of spinach or stir-fried vegetables.

Ingredients:

1 aubergine	2 tablespoons olive oil
1 onion, finely chopped	2 tomatoes, finely chopped
1 clove garlic, crushed	
4 button mushrooms, finely chopped	Salt & ground black pepper
	100g Emmental (or other hard cheese like Edam or Cheddar)

Method:

1) Preheat the oven to 350° F, 175° C, gas mark 4.

2) Cut the aubergine in two lengthways. Scoop out the flesh of the aubergine to leave two 'boats' made from the outside.

3) Chop the aubergine flesh finely and chop the other vegetables – onion, garlic, mushrooms and tomatoes.

4) Heat the oil in a wok, or large frying pan, until the olive oil is sizzling.

5) Stir-fry the onion and garlic for a couple of minutes alone before adding the mushrooms, aubergine and tomatoes. Season and then stir-fry everything until the vegetables are soft.

6) Pour the stir-fried vegetables into the aubergine boats.

7) Grate the Emmental on top.

8) Bake in the oven on, for approximately an hour, or until the cheese topping is crisp and brown.

TIP 1 – Can be a Phase 1 dish, if you leave out the cheese and mushrooms. This also makes the dish dairy-free.

Serves 2 – 1 boat each

Phase	Meal	V	C	H	Wheat-free	Dairy-free
(1 &) 2	Fat	✓	Can be	✓	✓	Can be

Butternut Squash Curry

This is the most luxurious Phase 1 dish possible, as it uses creamed coconut for flavouring. Creamed coconut is non-dairy and coconut oil has natural anti-Candida properties.

Ingredients:

2 tablespoons olive oil	500ml vegetable stock
3 onions, finely chopped	100g block of creamed coconut
4 cloves garlic, crushed	
2 teaspoons each of turmeric, cumin, paprika, coriander, chilli powder, curry powder (medium or hot depending on your preference)	1kg of mixed vegetables (cauliflower, courgettes, broccoli, carrots etc) chopped into 2cm cubes
	1 butternut squash, peeled
2 x 400ml tins of chopped tomatoes	deseeded and cut into 2cm squares

Method:

1) Heat the olive oil in a large saucepan and then gently fry the onions and garlic until soft.

2) Add the spices and gently fry for 1-2 minutes.

3) Add the tomatoes and vegetable stock and bring to the boil. Simmer for 5 minutes and then remove it from the heat and allow the mixture to cool slightly.

4) Using a hand blender, blend the mixture until smooth.

5) Return the mixture to the heat and stir in the creamed coconut block until it is completely dissolved.

6) You now have a delicious curry sauce to which you can add all the vegetables. Put the lid on the saucepan and simmer gently until the vegetables are cooked to your liking (approximately 30 minutes).

TIP 1 – Serve with brown rice, for a carb meal.

TIP 2 – Serve with chicken (and no carbs) for a chicken curry fat meal.

TIP 3 – This can be eaten on its own as a vegetable soup, or with wholemeal bread, as a carb meal.

Serves 4-6

Phase	Meal	V	C	H	Wheat-free	Dairy-free
1 & 2	Either	✓	✓	✓	✓	✓

Cheese Sauce

This sauce can be used to make either cauliflower cheese, or cheesy leeks, or any other cheese and vegetable dish. The recipe below uses cauliflower but pour the sauce over any vegetable you fancy. This also goes surprisingly well with white fish, if you fancy a non-Vegetarian meal.

Ingredients:

1 cauliflower, quartered, or 4 leeks, sliced or 4 white fish steaks 240ml milk	1 egg, whisked 100g Cheddar cheese, grated

Method:

1) For cauliflower cheese, or cheesy leeks, part cook the vegetables by lightly boiling or steaming them. Then place them in an oven-proof dish. For a white fish dish, brush the bottom of the oven-proof dish with olive oil and then place the fish steaks on top.

2) In a saucepan, bring the milk to the boil then turn off the heat. Allow the milk to cool for 2 minutes then mix in the whisked egg.

3) Add the grated cheese and stir continuously until the cheese has melted and you have a thick sauce.

4) Pour over the cauliflower, leeks or fish, sprinkle with a little grated cheese and place in the oven, 350° F, 175° C, gas mark 4, for 20-30 minutes. Serve hot.

TIP 1 – Serve the sauce with asparagus for a great fat starter.

TIP 2 – Sprinkle some fresh parsley, on top of the dish, just before serving, for a splash of colour and added taste.

TIP 3 – This also works really well with broccoli, instead of, or as well as, cauliflower.

Serves 4

Phase	Meal	V	C	H	Wheat-free	Dairy-free
2	Fat	Can be	✓	✓	✓	

Char Grilled Vegetables

If you leave out the balsamic and pine nuts, this makes a great Phase 1 recipe – a real bonus for Vegetarians, who can struggle in Phase 1.

Ingredients:

Olive oil for brushing a baking tray	Broccoli florets
	Peppers, any colours, sliced
1kg of mixed vegetables. The following work really well:	Carrots, peeled & sliced
	Parsnips, peeled & sliced
Aubergine, sliced with skin on	Butternut Squash, sliced with skin left on
Courgette, sliced with skin on	Balsamic Vinegar (optional)
Onions, peeled & sliced	Pine nuts & Parmesan (optional)

Method:

1) Preheat the oven to 350° F, 175° C, gas mark 4.

2) Brush a baking tray with olive oil.

3) Place the sliced vegetables on the baking tray and brush the vegetables with olive oil.

4) Roast them in the oven until the vegetables are charred around the edges and soft to a fork touch (approximately 30 minutes). (Note the parsnips and butternut squash will be soft in the middle but very crispy on the outside – you have just made healthy chips).

5) Flavour with balsamic vinegar (not in Phase 1, or if you have Candida) or extra olive oil if desired.

6) Add a few pine nuts and/or a small grating of Parmesan cheese for extra taste.

TIP 1 – Go easy on, or leave out, the butternut squash if you are very carbohydrate sensitive.

TIP 2 – Leave out the vinegar if you suffer from Candida.

Serves 4

Phase	Meal	V	C	H	Wheat-free	Dairy-free
1 & 2	Either	✓	Can be	✓	✓	✓

Vegetable Kebabs

Vegetable kebabs can be done with the same vegetables on a skewer, on a barbeque, or roasted in the oven.

Chef's Salad ☙

This is a base recipe – be your own chef and add in whatever you want – celeriac, beetroot, green beans – the more colour and vitamins the better.

Ingredients:

4 eggs (optional)	4 sticks celery
Diced cubes of ham, chicken & other cold meat	4 spring onions
	Red & green pepper strips
Diced cubes of hard cheese	1 carrot, grated
1 iceberg lettuce	Olive oil or another dressing
24 cherry tomatoes	Salt & ground black pepper
1 cucumber	

Method:

1) Hard-boil the eggs (place them in a saucepan of boiling water for 5-10 minutes, depending on how hard you like the yolks).

2) Dice the meat and cheese.

3) Chop the lettuce up quite finely and cover 4 plates with it. Slice the cherry tomatoes in two and place them around the edge of each plate.

4) Slice the cucumber, celery, spring onions and sprinkle these over the lettuce; add the pepper strips and grated carrot.

5) Quarter the hard-boiled eggs and arrange them on each plate. Add the meat and cheese cubes.

6) Add dressing to taste – olive oil is perfect.

TIP 1 – Can be a Phase 1 dish, if you leave out the cheese. This also makes the dish dairy-free.

TIP 2 – Can be a Vegetarian dish, if you leave out the meat.

Serves 4

Phase	Meal	V	C	H	Wheat-free	Dairy-free
(1 &) 2	Fat	Can be	✓	✓	✓	Can be

Egg & Asparagus Bake ♦

Use green beans or broccoli, instead of asparagus, if the latter is out of season.

Ingredients:

24 asparagus spears	100g grated Parmesan or "*Grana Padano*" cheese
4 tablespoons unsalted butter, melted	
4 eggs	Salt & ground black pepper

Method:

1) Pre-heat the oven to 400° F, 200° C, gas mark 6.

2) Steam the asparagus until tender and place evenly across the bottom of an oven-proof dish.

3) Whisk, or hand-beat, the eggs with the melted butter and pour the mixture over the asparagus.

4) Sprinkle the grated cheese over everything evenly and season with a dash of salt and ground black pepper.

5) Bake in the oven until the eggs are set and the cheese is golden brown – about 8-10 minutes.

Serves 4

Phase	Meal	V	C	H	Wheat-free	Dairy-free
2	Fat	✓	✓	✓	✓	

Four Cheese Salad ⏳

Try eating salads almost every day, even in the winter, as the goodness found in a large plate of raw vegetables is hard to beat. In the winter, combine salads with a warm soup and you will find this compensates for the chill of the salad.

Ingredients:

1 iceberg lettuce	200g cottage cheese
24 cherry tomatoes	50-75g per person of various cheese options (Cheddar, Edam, Emmental, Feta, Parmesan all work well), cubed
1 cucumber, diced	
4 sticks celery, diced	
1 red pepper, deseeded & diced	
Sprinkling of pine nuts (optional)	Salt & ground black pepper
Olive oil, or balsamic, or our French salad dressing	

Method:

1) Chop the lettuce up quite finely and cover 4 plates with it.

2) Slice the cherry tomatoes in two and place them around the edge of each plate.

3) Dice the cucumber, celery and pepper and sprinkle this over the lettuce (sprinkle a few pine nuts on too if you like these).

4) Add your chosen dressing over the salad base.

5) Place 50g, or so, of cottage cheese in the middle of each plate.

6) Add cubes of cheese (approx 1cm cube) to taste around the cottage cheese. Feta with balsamic and cottage cheese goes really well together, so do Cheddar, Emmental, Parmesan and cottage cheese.

Serves 4

Phase	Meal	V	C	H	Wheat-free	Dairy-free
2	Fat	✓	✓	✓	✓	

Fruit Platters ⚍ ☺

Take care to stick to just 1-2 portions of fruit a day, if you have Candida and/or Hypoglycaemia.

Ingredients:

A good selection of ripe, fresh, fruit in season (washed) e.g.: Apples; Pears, Oranges, Grapes, Nectarines, Peaches, Melon	Low fat Natural Live Yoghurt (optional) Low fat cottage cheese (optional)

Method:

1) Get an oversized plate/platter (a normal plate will be fine if you don't have a giant one).

2) Get peeling, chopping and slicing. Leave any edible skins on and chop all the fruit so that you just have to dive in with fingers and enjoy. This is a really satisfying meal and seems a lot more filling than when you just eat pieces of fruit on their own. You can add a couple of spoonfuls of low fat cottage cheese or low fat Natural Live Yoghurt in the middle of the platter for a filling dip.

Tropical Fruit Platter:

Pineapple, mango, melon, paw paw, papaya, banana, sharon fruit, star fruit, kiwi fruit and grapes – whatever you can find in the supermarket.

Berry Fruit Platter:

Strawberries, raspberries, blueberries and blackberries – again whatever you can find.

Stone Fruit Platter:

Nectarines, peaches, plums and apricots.

Citrus Fruit Platter:

Orange segments, grapefruit segments, kumquats, satsumas and clementines.

Staple Fruit Platter:

Available all year round – sliced apples, sliced pears, grapes and bananas.

Phase	Meal	V	C	H	Wheat-free	Dairy-free
2	Carb	✓	(✓)	(✓)	✓	Can be

Omelettes (No Milk)

Ingredients:

2-3 eggs	Knob of butter
_ teaspoon mixed herbs	Ground black pepper

Method:

1) Crack 2 or 3 eggs per person into a mixing bowl and beat with a fork, or an electric whisk, until fluffy.

2) Add about _ teaspoon of mixed herbs and some freshly ground black pepper.

3) Melt a knob of butter in a frying pan and add the whisked eggs.

4) Cook slowly until the mixture becomes firm. (You can tilt the pan to move the mixture around to make sure it covers the pan but don't stir it or you will end up with scrambled eggs).

This can be served with a mixed salad for a main meal.

For a flavoured Omelette, add some of your favourite ingredients to the whisked eggs before pouring them into the frying pan. The classic options are ham, cheese and mushrooms (no mushrooms for Candida).

Serves 1

Phase	Meal	V	C	H	Wheat-free	Dairy-free
1 & 2	Fat	Can be	✓	✓	✓	✓

Paella (Seafood or Bean)

You can put seafood in for a Phase 1 dish – or leave the seafood out for a Phase 1 Vegetarian dish. In Phase 2, when you don't mix fats and carbs, use beans instead of seafood, to make it a carb meal.

Ingredients:

350g (dry weight) brown rice	2 'beef' tomatoes, chopped
2 tablespoons olive oil	Salt & ground black pepper
2 cloves garlic, crushed	_ teaspoon turmeric
2 onions, finely chopped	_ teaspoon oregano
1 stick celery, finely chopped	2 tablespoons parsley, chopped
1 green pepper, deseeded & diced	100g button mushrooms (leave out for Phase 1)
1 aubergine, diced	200g seafood (Phase 1) OR 100g tin red kidney beans (Phase 2)
2 carrots, peeled & diced	

Method:

1) Boil a kettle and put the brown rice in a pan of boiling water to cook. Chop all the vegetables (do this in fewer than 10-15 minutes and then the timing will be perfect for the stir-fry being done at the same time as the rice).

2) Heat the oil in a wok, or large frying pan.

3) Stir-fry the garlic, onions, celery, pepper, aubergine and carrots for approximately 10 minutes, until the carrots are starting to soften.

4) Add the tomatoes and mushrooms and cook for a further 5 minutes.

5) Drain the rice and add it to the vegetable mixture. Add the kidney beans too and the seasoning, turmeric and oregano.

6) Cook on a very low heat for a further 15 minutes.

7) Serve with the chopped Parsley on top as garnish.

TIP 1 – Leave out the seafood and mushrooms and this can be suitable for Phase 1 and Candida – great for Vegetarians who struggle in Phase 1.

Serves 4

Seafood version (no mushrooms)

Phase	Meal	V	C	H	Wheat-free	Dairy-free
1	Mixed	✓	✓	✓	✓	✓

Bean version

Phase	Meal	V	C	H	Wheat-free	Dairy-free
2	Carb	✓	✓	✓	✓	✓

Ratatouille ☙

This recipe is great with fish, or it can be served with pasta instead of plain tomato sauce. It also goes really well with Quorn and Tofu.

Ingredients:

6 tablespoons olive oil	1 green pepper, deseeded & chopped
2 aubergines, diced in 2cm squares	1 clove garlic, finely chopped
2 courgettes, cut into batons	400g tin chopped tomatoes
2 onions, finely sliced	Salt & ground black pepper
1 red pepper, deseeded & chopped	

Method:

1) Heat the olive oil in a wok, or large frying pan, until the olive oil is warm.

2) Cook the aubergines until they are browned, stirring regularly to brown them all over. Transfer them to a casserole dish.

3) Cook the courgette batons in the wok/pan until they are browned, stirring regularly to brown them all over. Transfer them to the casserole dish.

4) Put the onions in the wok/pan and cook them for 2-3 minutes.

5) Add the peppers and garlic and cook for a further 3-4 minutes, until soft.

6) Transfer the onions, peppers and garlic to the casserole dish with the aubergines and courgettes.

7) Pour the tin of chopped tomatoes on top. Season to taste.

8) Put a lid on the casserole dish and cook in the ingredients in a low oven 325° F, 165° C, gas mark 3 for approximately 45 minutes.

Serve with a baked potato, wholemeal sugar-free bread or brown rice for a carb meal, or with fish or meat for a fat meal

Serves 4

Phase	Meal	V	C	H	Wheat-free	Dairy-free
1 & 2	Either	✓	✓	✓	✓	✓

Roasted Vegetables with Pine Nuts & Parmesan

This is a really simple and colourful dish that is especially nice in the winter when the vegetables are in season. There are a few nuts and a bit of cheese in this recipe, but not enough to make any difference to your weight loss and they really add to the flavour.

Ingredients:

2 tablespoons olive oil	200g mixed salad leaves
2 onions, quartered	Sprinkling of Parmesan cheese, grated (optional)
1 clove garlic, crushed	
1kg of mixed vegetables, cubed (Use butternut squash, aubergines & courgettes etc)	A sprinkling of pine nuts (optional)
	Balsamic vinegar (leave out for Candida)
1 red pepper, deseeded & diced	

Method:

1) Preheat the oven to 400° F, 200° C, gas mark 6.

2) In a wok, or large frying pan, heat the oil and gently fry the onions and garlic for 2 minutes; then add all the other vegetables and stir-fry for a further 2 minutes.

3) Put the vegetables in a large oven-proof dish and roast in the oven for 30 minutes, stirring half way through.

4) To serve, place a small amount of mixed green lettuce in an open, pasta type bowl and spoon on the roasted vegetables. Sprinkle with the grated Parmesan cheese and pine nuts and place under a very hot grill for 2 minutes just to melt the cheese.

Dribble a small amount of balsamic vinegar around the edge of the bowl and serve immediately.

TIP 1 – Go for the lower glycaemic index vegetables, like courgettes, rather than butternut squash, if you are very carbohydrate sensitive.

TIP 2 – Leave out the vinegar to be suitable for Candida.

Serves 4

Phase	Meal	V	C	H	Wheat-free	Dairy-free
2	Either	✓	Can be	✓	✓	Can be

Roast Chicken with Garlic & Lemon ☺

You can cook chicken in the oven, in its own juices, with absolutely nothing else, but for even more flavour, stuff it with cloves of garlic and fresh lemons as follows.

Ingredients:

1 whole chicken	6-8 cloves garlic
	1 whole lemon

Method:

1) Preheat the oven to 350° F, 175° C, gas mark 4.

2) Allow 6-8 cloves of garlic and 1 whole lemon cut in quarters, for a medium sized chicken.

3) Remove the giblets and then stuff the garlic cloves and lemon quarters into the inside of the chicken.

4) Cook 'up-side-down' for the first 30 minutes for the juices to penetrate the breast meat and then turn over.

5) Cook for a further 30-60 minutes.

Serve with a selection of vegetables in the winter or a mixed salad in the summer.

Serves 4

Phase	Meal	V	C	H	Wheat-free	Dairy-free
1 & 2	Fat		✓	✓	✓	✓

Roast Leg of Lamb with Rosemary & Vegetables

This is the lamb equivalent of the simple chicken dish.

Ingredients:

1 leg of lamb 6-8 cloves garlic	Rosemary (fresh sprig if possible)

Method:

1) Preheat the oven to 400° F, 200° C, gas mark 6.

2) Place the leg of lamb in a large roasting dish and sprinkle with rosemary (fresh if possible).

3) Add a handful of garlic cloves (unpeeled) and pop the lot in the oven and roast until cooked to your liking.

4) As a guide, allow the following cooking times:

- Pink: 10 minutes for every 450g plus 20 minutes;

- Medium: 15 minutes for every 450g plus 20 minutes;

- Well done: 20 minutes for every 450g plus 20 minutes.

Serve with a selection of freshly cooked vegetables or stir-fried vegetables. The garlic cooked this way becomes sweet and can be eaten with the meat.

Serves 4

Phase	Meal	V	C	H	Wheat-free	Dairy-free
1 & 2	Fat		✓	✓	✓	✓

Salade Niçoise/Salmon Niçoise ⚉

This is one of the healthiest and simplest main meals of all. The classic recipe has diced potatoes on top, but leave these out to keep the carbs away from this fat meal.

Ingredients:

150g green beans	4 Char grilled tuna steaks or 400g tinned tuna (or salmon steaks or tinned salmon for Salmon Niçoise)
4 eggs	
1 iceberg lettuce	
24 cherry tomatoes	Olive oil or another dressing
1 cucumber	
	Salt & ground black pepper

Method:

1) Chop the green beans into lengths of 3-4cm long. Cook them in boiling water until they are as soft or as crunchy as you like them.

2) Hard-boil the eggs (place them in a saucepan of boiling water for 5-10 minutes, depending on how hard you like the yolks).

3) Chop the lettuce up quite finely and cover 4 plates with it. Slice the cherry tomatoes in two and place them around the edge of each plate.

4) Dice the cucumber and sprinkle this over the lettuce; add the cooked green beans when they have cooled.

5) Quarter the hard-boiled eggs and arrange them on each plate.

6) Add dressing to taste – olive oil is perfect.

7) Place the char grilled tuna steaks (cook raw tuna on the barbeque, or in a frying pan, or just place it under a normal grill) or the tinned tuna in the middle of the plate.

TIP 1 – You can cook the green beans in the same pan as the eggs but this can discolour the green beans. Two pans and bright green beans or one pan and the possibility of slightly grey beans – the choice is yours.

TIP 2 – Add anchovies for garnish and authenticity.

Serves 4

Phase	Meal	V	C	H	Wheat-free	Dairy-free
1 & 2	Fat		✓	✓	✓	✓

Scrambled Eggs (No Milk)

Ingredients:

2 eggs	Knob of butter

Method:

1) Crack 2 eggs per person into a mixing bowl and beat with a fork, or an electric whisk, until fluffy.

2) Melt a knob of butter in a frying pan and add the whisked eggs.

3) Continually stir the eggs in the pan (with a wooden spoon) until they become the consistency that you like. The longer you cook them the firmer they will get.

Serves 1

Phase	Meal	V	C	H	Wheat-free	Dairy-free
1 & 2	Fat	✓	✓	✓	✓	✓

Scrambled Eggs (With Milk)

As above, but add the same volume as the eggs, in milk, when you first crack the eggs into a bowl.

Stir-Fry Vegetables

Ingredients:

Any vegetables you like. E.g. Onion Garlic Baby sweet corn Mange tout	Bean sprouts Peppers Courgettes Carrots Green beans

Method:

1) Clean and chop any mixture of vegetables into bite size pieces (carrot batons, green beans in 3-4cm lengths, 3-4cm strips of coloured peppers, roughly chopped onions, crushed garlic, baby sweet corn cut into two, mange tout pieces, bean sprouts, water chestnuts etc).

2) Put the onion and peppers into a wok, or large frying pan, and cook them until they brown on the edges (you can use a tablespoon or two of olive oil, but none is necessary).

3) Throw in the garlic and then cook for approximately 30-60 seconds.

4) Add the rest of the vegetables. Stir-fry for 2-3 minutes.

5) Then add a soup ladle full of tap water and cook until the water is evaporated and serve. This seals in all the flavour and the goodness of the vegetables.

Phase	Meal	V	C	H	Wheat-free	Dairy-free
1 & 2	Either	✓	✓	✓	✓	✓

Stuffed Peppers/Tomatoes

This can be done with either peppers or large tomatoes. The recipe below uses peppers as an example. Use multi-coloured peppers if you are cooking this for several people, so that you get a real assortment of colour.

Ingredients:

100g brown rice	1 clove garlic, crushed
1 litre vegetable stock	4 mushrooms, finely chopped (leave out for Phase 1)
4 peppers (red, green or yellow)	
	1 teaspoon mixed herbs
1 tablespoon olive oil	Freshly ground black pepper
1 onion, finely chopped	

Method:

1) Preheat the oven to 350° F, 175° C, gas mark 4.

2) Cook the brown rice in the vegetable stock for approximately 30 minutes.

3) Meanwhile, prepare the peppers by slicing the tops off (keeping them intact) and scoop out the seeds from the middle. The idea is to make a 'bowl' with a 'lid', out of the peppers, to stuff the other ingredients into.

4) Approximately 5 minutes before the rice is cooked, gently fry the onion, garlic and mushrooms in the olive oil until soft.

5) Add the herbs and stir in the cooked brown rice. Add some freshly ground black pepper and stuff the mixture into the prepared peppers.

6) Replace the top on the peppers and place them in an oven-proof dish. Bake for approximately 20-30 minutes.

Serve them with ratatouille, or on their own.

TIP 1 – Leave out the mushrooms, or use another vegetable (e.g. courgettes) instead, and this can be suitable for Phase 1 and Candida.

Serves 4

Phase	Meal	V	C	H	Wheat-free	Dairy-free
1 & 2	Carb	✓	Can be	✓	✓	✓

Vegetarian Chilli

Vegetarian chilli is another classic recipe that every household cook should be able to dish up at any time. This is a really filling dish and great for re-heating for quick meals. As the beans provide protein, this can be eaten as a meal in itself, if you don't have time to do rice or a baked potato to go with it.

Ingredients:

2 tablespoons olive oil	400g tin of unsweetened kidney beans, drained
2 onions, finely chopped	400g tin chopped tomatoes
1 red pepper, deseeded & chopped	2 chillies, deseeded & sliced
1 clove garlic, crushed	Chilli powder to taste (somewhere between 2 and 4 teaspoons)
1.5kg of mixed vegetables cut into 2cm cubes. Use carrots, courgette, cauliflower, broccoli, leeks – anything you like	

Method:

1) In a large saucepan or wok, heat the oil and gently fry the onions until soft.

2) Add the pepper and garlic and fry for a further 3-4 minutes.

3) Then add all the mixed vegetables, including the kidney beans, tinned tomatoes and chillies and give it all a good stir.

4) Stir in the chilli powder and then put the lid on the pan. Bring to the boil and then reduce to simmering point and cook for 20-30 minutes, or until the vegetables are cooked to your liking.

TIP 1 – Leave out the mushrooms to make this recipe suitable for Candida.

Serve with brown rice, or a crispy baked potato.

Serves 4-6

Phase	Meal	V	C	H	Wheat-free	Dairy-free
2	Carb	✓	✓	✓	✓	✓

Part 8
Appendices

Appendix 1 – Glossary of Terms

Blood Glucose Level – our blood has to keep a certain level of 'glucose' at all times. If it goes above or below the safe levels of glucose, this can be really serious – even life threatening.

Candida – is a yeast, which lives in all of us, and is normally kept under control by our immune system and other bacteria in our body. It usually lives in the digestive system. Candida has no useful purpose. If it stays in balance, it causes no harm. If it multiplies out of control, it can create havoc with our health.

Diabetes – this is the condition that someone has if their pancreas does not produce any, or enough, insulin to return their blood glucose level back to normal after they have eaten a carbohydrate. Before the drug insulin was developed, Diabetics had to follow a diet with virtually no carbohydrate, to ensure that their blood glucose level stayed within the normal range.

Food Intolerance – means, quite simply, not being able to tolerate a particular food. Food Intolerance develops when you have too much of a food, too often, and your body just gets to the point where it can't cope with that food any longer. Food Intolerance can make a person feel horribly unwell.

Glycaemic Index – this is the measure of the effect of any food on blood glucose levels over a period of time. Glucose is the purest substance from which the body can get energy. The index uses the impact of pure glucose being consumed as '100' and then measures all other foods against this.

Hypoglycaemia – is literally a Greek translation from "*hypo*" meaning 'under', "*glykis*" meaning 'sweet' and "*emia*" meaning 'in the blood together'. The three bits all put together mean low blood sugar. Hypoglycaemia describes the state the body is in if your blood sugar levels are too low. When your blood sugar levels are too low, this is potentially life threatening and your body will try to get you to eat.

Insulin – is a hormone produced by the pancreas. When we eat a carbohydrate our body converts this into glucose and so the level of glucose in our blood rises. This is dangerous for the human body so we have this fantastic mechanism within the pancreas, which ensures that insulin is released from the pancreas to 'mop up' the excess glucose and to return our blood glucose level to normal.

Insulin resistance – this describes the situation where our bodies don't respond properly to the release of insulin. With insulin resistance, eating carbohydrates causes insulin to be released, but the body fails to use this insulin efficiently and, therefore, the carbohydrates get stored as more fat instead, adding to your weight problem further. It has been shown that 92% of people with Type II Diabetes have insulin resistance. (Type II Diabetes is the one developed by older people – not the one that teenagers tend to get very suddenly).

Syndrome X – is a term used by doctors to group together a number of conditions, which they have often seen together, in a patient. They have observed that people with insulin resistance are also highly likely to have: insulin resistance; raised blood fats; raised cholesterol; raised blood glucose levels; high blood pressure and so on. By looking at these conditions together they are able to treat the patient '.

Appendix 2 – Recommended Reading

Candida

Candida – a Twentieth Century Disease by Shirley Lorenzani (1986)

The Yeast Syndrome by John Parks Trowbridge MD and Morton Walker D.P.M. (1986)

Candida Albicans – Could Yeast be your problem? by Leon Chaitow (1987)

The Yeast Connection by William G. Crook MD (1983)

The Complete Candida Yeast Guidebook by Martin & Rona (2000)

Beat Candida by Gill Jacobs (1990)

Food Intolerance

Food Intolerance – What it is & How to cope with it by Robert Buist (1984)

5-day Allergy Relief System by Dr Marshall Mandell and Lynne Scanlon (1979)

The Allergy Handbook by Dr Keith Mumby (1988)

Allergies – Your Hidden Enemy? by Theron Randolph MD & Ralph W. Moss PhD (1981)

Not all in the Mind by Dr Richard Mackarness (1976)

The False Fat Diet by Elson M Haas MD & Cameron Stauth (2001)

The Complete Guide to Food Allergy and Intolerance by Dr Jonathan Brostoff & Linda Gamlin (1989)

Hypoglycaemia

Hypoglycaemia – The Disease your Doctor Won't Treat by Saunders & Ross (1980)

Low Blood glucose (Hypoglycaemia) The twentieth century Epidemic? by Martin L Budd (1983)

New low blood sugar & you by Carlton Fredericks (1985)

Appendix 3

Vitamins & Minerals

Recommended Daily Allowances (RDA'S), of foods and supplements has traditionally been set by government health bodies in the USA, UK, and Europe. In the USA, RDA stands for "Recommended Daily Dietary Allowance", which is established for each vitamin and mineral by the Food and Nutritional Board of the National Academy of Sciences and the Food and Drug Administration (FDA).

In the UK the Department of Health gave the RDA for vitamins A, C, and D, three of the B vitamins, and three minerals in 1979. However, in 1993, the European Union (EU) issued a directive on food labelling for its members, which included RDA's for twelve vitamins and six minerals.

Governments and food agencies are continually reviewing the RDA's. For the following two tables, we have used the 2004 EU RDA's given for twelve vitamins and six minerals. Where no RDA's have been given for Vitamin K and for the minerals: chromium; copper; manganese; potassium and selenium, we have taken the best recommendations from *The Thorsons Complete Guide to Vitamins & Minerals* – generally regarded as the vitamin and mineral bible.

Notation

RDA = Recommended Daily Allowance

mg = milligrams

µg = micrograms = 3.33 IU's (International Units)

Summary (Vitamins)

VITAMIN	NEEDED FOR?	RDA	BEST SOURCES?
A	Eyesight, growth, appetite & taste	800µg	Liver, butter, cheese, eggs, carrots
B1	Nervous system, digestion, muscles, heart	1.4mg	Liver, yeast, brown rice, whole-grains, peanuts
B2	Growth, skin, nails, hair, eyesight	1.6mg	Milk, liver, yeast, cheese, fish
B3	Energy conversion, building red blood cells	1.8mg	Liver, whole-grains, eggs, avocado, fish, meat, peanuts
B5	Energy conversion, fatigue, stress	6mg	Fish, liver, chicken, yeast, whole-grains, milk, cheese, eggs
B6	Blood, nerves, mental health	2mg	Fish, bananas, pork, whole-grains
B8 (Biotin)	Energy conversion; skin, hair, nerves & bone marrow	150µg	Dried brewers yeast, yeast, eggs, whole grains, corn
B9 (Folic Acid)	Blood formation & resisting infection	300µg	Carrots, yeast, liver, apricots, pulses, green vegetables

B12	The basis of all body cells	2µg	Fish, liver, beef, pork, milk, cheese – only animal foods
C	Absorbing iron; resisting infection; controlling cholesterol	60mg	Fruits & vegetables
D	Bones & muscles	5µg	Cod liver oil, oily fish, eggs, sunlight
E	Healthy blood & anti-blood clotting	10mg	Nuts, soya beans, olive oil, eggs, green vegetables
K	Blood clotting & bones	No EU RDA	Liver, egg yolk, green vegetables, cheese

Copies available on *www.theharcombediet.com*

Summary (Minerals)

MINERAL	NEEDED FOR?	RDA	BEST SOURCES?
Calcium	Bones & teeth	500mg	Milk, cheese, tinned fish, nuts, pulses
Chromium	Controlling blood glucose level	No EU RDA (200µg optional)	Egg yolks, dried brewers yeast, beef, cheese, liver
Copper	Bones, skin, hair; resisting infection	No EU RDA (2mg optional)	Liver, shell fish, dried brewers yeast, olives. Also copper pipes & containers
Iron	Carrying oxygen to red blood cells	14mg	Dried brewers yeast, liver, kidney, cocoa, dried fruits
Iodine	Thyroid function	150µg	Kelp, haddock, whiting & small amounts in other fish
Magnesium	Energy production, body growth & repair	300mg	Soya beans, dried brewers yeast, nuts, whole grains
Manganese	Growth & nervous system	No EU RDA (2mg optional)	Whole grains, nuts, pulses

Phosphorus	Bones & teeth, activates the B complex for energy	800mg	Yeast extract, dried brewers yeast, canned fish
Potassium	Energy production, water balance, body cell health	No EU RDA (2g optional)	Soy flour, bananas, dried fruits, salads, vegetables, nuts, fruit, brown rice
Selenium	Liver, heart, hair, skin, eyes, fighting infection	No EU RDA (200µg optional)	Kidneys & liver, fish & shellfish, whole grains
Zinc	Growth, insulin balance	15mg	Oysters, liver, dried brewers yeast, shellfish, meat, cheese, fish

Copies available on *www.theharcombediet.com*

About The Author...

Zoë's passion is now her vocation. Zoë spends her time researching and writing about obesity, diets and weight loss and she works exclusively in this field. She is author of the best selling book *The Harcombe Diet: Stop Counting Calories and Start Losing Weight* which was the follow-up to *Why do you overeat? When all you want is to be slim.*

The result of 20 years' research into the causes of overeating, Zoë's books go against traditional diets and are the first to address the three fundamental medical conditions that cause food cravings and therefore the compulsion to overeat. This understanding has helped thousands of people lose weight quickly, easily and healthily through The Harcombe Diet approach.

During her teenage years Zoë suffered from both anorexia and bulimia, which she battled for several years before becoming the first person from her state school to graduate from Cambridge University. The early years of her career were then spent fighting food cravings to rival any drug addiction.

Despite her illnesses and ongoing struggle with food, Zoë developed her career and achieved a number of high powered positions in the management consultancy, consumer goods, pharmaceuticals and telecommunications industries for blue chip organisations including Mars and SmithKline Beecham.

During her 20's, Zoë suffered from all three of the medical conditions detailed in her books but no longer suffers from any of them and knows how to make sure they, and food cravings, never return.

Zoë has now been free from food addiction for over 10 years and decided to put her years of experience and research onto paper, creating the heart-felt, revolutionary diet book, *Why do you overeat?*, followed by *Stop Counting Calories & Start Losing Weight* and the accompanying recipe book.

She is now a full-time diet guru with a Diploma in Diet and Nutrition and a Diploma in Clinical Weight Management and spends her time advising clients, writing for newspapers and magazines, appearing as a diet expert on TV and radio, undertaking more research, and inspiring women and men world-wide.

Zoë lives with her husband, Andy, a rescue dog and cat in the beautiful Welsh countryside. She is a member of The National Obesity Forum, The Federation of Holistic Therapists, Mensa and The Chocolate Society.

To find out more about Zoë and/or The Harcombe Diet, please visit:

www.zoeharcombe.com

www.theharcombediet.com

For more recipes

Stop Counting Calories & Start Losing Weight

The Harcombe Diet Recipe Book

Packed with full flavour recipes for healthier eating and effortless weight-loss.

Zoë Harcombe, author of *The Harcombe Diet* and trained chef, Rachel McGuinness, have teamed up to produce over 250 delicious and healthy recipes to help people *Stop Counting Calories and Start Losing Weight*. The partnership has produced a fantastic selection of recipes that are nutritious, delicious and easy to cook. The recipes feature real food, real ingredients, no manufactured fats, minimal sugar (if any) – just health and taste – which is what the diet is all about.

Available as an ebook on www.theharcombediet.com

Index

alcohol, v, ix, 21, 22, 55, 60, 64, 65, 72, 88, 103, 117, 168, 191, 192, 193, 215, 261, 289

allergy, 68, 70, 71, 75, 83, 86, 95, 100, 124

Anorexia, 173, 177, 180, 181

antibiotics, 51, 52, 57, 65, 67, 159, 232, 279

Atkins, iv, 8, 10, 17, 23

avocados, 208

Biotin, 53, 64, 278, 279, 336

Blood Glucose, 4, 55, 60, 72, 93, 330

BMI, 28, 29, 30, 31

bulimia, 173, 174, 177, 178, 180, 181, 188

caffeine, 55, 60, 72, 93, 146, 147, 167, 192, 243, 259, 260

cereal, 10, 23, 39, 41, 42, 44, 70, 74, 80, 81, 102, 112, 113, 114, 115, 119, 123, 127, 136, 139, 141, 144, 166, 175, 201, 207, 209, 240, 244, 246, 254, 267, 272, 276, 284

chips, 19, 119, 120, 165, 174, 201, 206, 242, 245, 247, 250, 287, 302

chromium, 235, 281, 335

coffee, 70, 74, 103, 111, 113, 115, 117, 146, 167, 168, 259, 260, 261, 263, 285

constipation, 10, 54, 71, 263

corn flour, 242

cream, vi, 80, 81, 89, 123, 124, 130, 136, 138, 156, 157, 158, 160, 164, 165, 174, 178, 195, 198, 242, 255

crème fresh, 209, 242

Diabetes, 32, 51, 52, 57, 65, 88, 92, 95, 264, 266, 330, 331

Diabetic, 52, 88

diet coke, 260

exercise, ix, 7, 8, 18, 19, 32, 156, 194, 227

Flexis, 17, 109, 134

food addiction, 47, 73, 164, 176, 177, 183, 184, 188, 190, 191, 192, 194, 195, 196, 198, 221, 222, 223, 233, 274, 291

Food Allergy, 5, 332

food family, 82, 83, 86, 160, 279

fromage frais, 209, 242

fruit, 4, 5, 10, 12, 16, 17, 21, 23, 39, 41, 44, 51, 57, 62, 63, 70, 103, 117, 118, 119, 121, 126, 127, 128, 131, 132, 135, 136, 138, 139, 140, 143, 148, 166, 168, 173, 176, 208, 209, 224, 226, 230, 235, 236, 238, 239, 243, 246, 247, 250, 256, 258, 263, 277, 278, 279, 283, 285, 286, 309, 339

GI, 12, 13, 14

Glycaemic Index, 12, 13, 330

grazing, 162

Herxheimer's' reaction, 107

honey, 81, 119, 121, 208

hormones, 51, 52, 57, 65, 159

hummus, 17, 209

Insulin, 4, 219, 266, 331

insulin resistance, 266, 267, 331

low calorie diet, 11, 46

lowest sugar fruits, 128

mascarpone cheese, 243

natural weight, 8, 15, 18, 29, 98, 118, 119, 129, 156, 157, 162, 163, 181, 200, 202, 218, 221, 262, 288

Newburgh and Johnson, 33

nuts, 54, 68, 81, 86, 122, 132, 137, 166, 210, 211, 302, 303, 307, 316, 338, 339

obesity, 2, 3, 18, 31, 32, 35, 36, 37, 52, 185

pasta, 10, 14, 16, 17, 21, 57, 70, 74, 76, 80, 81, 82, 118, 119, 120, 122, 123, 125, 137, 142, 145, 157, 158, 159, 164, 178, 237, 243, 244, 253, 255, 263, 272, 277, 279, 281, 282, 283, 285, 288, 295, 314, 316

Planners, 17, 111, 112, 114, 140, 143

potatoes, 16, 89, 101, 117, 119, 120, 124, 130, 139, 160, 165, 168, 199, 242, 245, 254, 256, 277, 282, 287, 288, 320

pregnancy, 71, 270, 271

preservatives, 62, 257

preserves, 136, 258

pulses, 65, 126, 244, 253, 336, 338

Quorn, 123, 124, 137, 160, 212, 253, 295, 314

seeds, 110, 131, 132, 141, 144, 206, 210, 211, 324

smoked, 17, 100, 113, 135, 136, 246

South Beach Diet, 11, 12

soya milk, 208

steroids, 51, 52, 57, 65, 67, 159

stock cube, 246

successful diet, 7, 8, 12, 14, 15, 98, 158

sugar-free gum, 241

sweet corn, 80, 247, 323

sweet potatoes, 210

sweeteners, 207, 241, 242, 258

Syndrome X, 266, 267, 331

The Zone, 11, 12

Tofu, 81, 101, 110, 111, 114, 115, 117, 123, 124, 141, 160, 168, 211, 212, 253, 295, 314

Vegan, 20, 102, 212

Vegetarian, ix, 19, 20, 101, 102, 114, 123, 124, 137, 142, 143, 145, 164, 211, 244, 253, 284, 287, 294, 305, 312, 326

vinegar, 51, 62, 126, 136, 176, 186, 188, 229, 242, 248, 302, 303, 316, 317

Why do you overeat, iii, 2, 176, 264

LaVergne, TN USA
28 February 2010
174444LV00002B/1/P